The Massachusetts General Hospital Approach to Transcatheter Arterialization of the Deep Veins for Advanced Limb Salvage

Anahita Dua · Sara Rose-Sauld
Lindsey Ferraro · Erin Sweeney
Editors

The Massachusetts General Hospital Approach to Transcatheter Arterialization of the Deep Veins for Advanced Limb Salvage

Protocols and Procedures

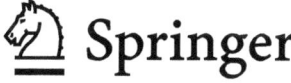 Springer

Editors
Anahita Dua
Vascular Surgery
Massachusetts General Hospital/
Harvard Medical School
Boston, MA, USA

Lindsey Ferraro
Massachusetts General Hospital
Boston, MA, USA

Sara Rose-Sauld
Massachusetts General Hospital
Boston, MA, USA

Erin Sweeney
Massachusetts General Hospital
Boston, MA, USA

ISBN 978-3-031-37512-5   ISBN 978-3-031-37510-1   (eBook)
https://doi.org/10.1007/978-3-031-37510-1

This Springer imprint is published by the registered company Springer Nature Switzerland AG
The registered company address is: Gewerbestrasse 11, 6330 Cham, Switzerland

We dedicate this textbook to all of our incredible patients past, present, and future.

Contents

Part I Patient Identification

1 **Selecting the Correct Patient Candidate** 3
Anahita Dua, Sara Rose-Sauld, and Lindsey Ferraro

2 **Evaluating the Angiogram** 7
Anahita Dua, Sara Rose-Sauld, and Lindsey Ferraro

3 **Preprocedural Wound Considerations** 11
Anahita Dua, Sara Rose-Sauld, and Lindsey Ferraro

4 **Explaining TADV to the Patient and Family** 31
Anahita Dua, Sara Rose-Sauld, and Lindsey Ferraro

Part II Patient Preparation

5 **Duplex Pedal Mapping for Case Preparation** 37
Anahita Dua, Sara Rose-Sauld, and Lindsey Ferraro

6 **Preoperative Optimization of the Patient** 45
Anahita Dua, Gaurav Parmar, Sara Rose-Sauld,
and Lindsey Ferraro

Part III Procedure and Acute Post-operative Care

7 **Overview of TADV and Required Equipment** 53
Anahita Dua, Sara Rose-Sauld, and Lindsey Ferraro

8   Pedal Venous Access 57
     Anahita Dua, Sara Rose-Sauld, and Lindsey Ferraro

9   Procedural Steps 61
     Anahita Dua, Sara Rose-Sauld, and Lindsey Ferraro

10   Immediate Postoperative Care. 87
     Anahita Dua, Sara Rose-Sauld, and Lindsey Ferraro

11   Post-TADV Care Plan. 91
     Anahita Dua, Sara Rose-Sauld, and Lindsey Ferraro

Part IV   Post-procedure Care and Maintenance

12   Imaging the TADV Circuit. 97
     Lindsey Ferraro, Sara Rose-Sauld, and Anahita Dua

13   Circuit Maintenance and Optimization 105
     Anahita Dua, Sara Rose-Sauld, and Lindsey Ferraro

14   Wound Care. 117
     Anahita Dua, Sara Rose-Sauld, and Lindsey Ferraro

**15   TADV and Beyond: Postoperative Care of
     the Patient with Forefoot Amputation**. 121
     Nikolaos Zacharias

Index. 133

Editors and Contributors

About the Editors

Anahita Dua MD MS MBA FACS, is an Associate Professor of Surgery at Harvard Medical School and a vascular surgeon at the Massachusetts General Hospital. She is the director of the vascular lab, co-director of the Peripheral Artery Disease Center and Limb Evaluation and Amputation Prevention program (LEAPP), associate director of the wound care program, and director of clinical research. She specializes in advanced endovascular and open techniques for the care of patients with peripheral arterial disease (PAD), diabetic limb disease, aortic disease, carotid disease, thoracic outlet syndrome (TOS), and venous disease. She completed her vascular surgery fellowship at Stanford Hospital and her General Surgery residency at the Medical College of Wisconsin. She has completed a master's degree in trauma sciences, an MBA in Healthcare Management, a certificate in health economics and outcomes research as well as a certificate in drug and device development from MIT. She is nationally certified in advanced wound care and management. Dr. Dua has published over 170 peer-reviewed papers and has edited 5 vascular surgery medical textbooks. She serves on multiple national vascular surgery committees through the Society for Vascular Surgery and other vascular organizations.

Sara Rose-Sauld DPM, is a podiatrist at the Massachusetts General Hospital specializing in limb salvage for the diabetic foot. She serves in the Division of Foot and Ankle Surgery. Dr. Rose-Sauld completed her podiatry training at Palmetto General Hospital in Florida with a focus on reconstructive procedures and wound care. She is the head of podiatry services through the LEAPP limb salvage center.

Lindsey Ferraro MS, RDCS, RVT, is a Lead Vascular Technologist at the Vascular Lab at Massachusetts General Hospital and the Lead Vascular

Sonographer Liaison for the MGH LEAPP. Lindsey also works as the lead sonographer and consultant for vascular ultrasound research specializing in pedal access for critical limb ischemia. She is credentialed by the American Registry of Diagnostic Medical Sonography in Cardiac and Vascular Specialties. She has multiple published peer-reviewed articles and is an Ad-Hoc Editor for multiple papers. She received her Bachelor of Science Degree from Grand Valley State University in Medical Imaging and Radiation Sciences and a Master of Science Degree in Emergency Management/Crisis Management from Southern New Hampshire University. She also volunteers for various professional organizations such as the Society of Diagnostic Medical Sonography and the American Red Cross Disaster Action Team.

Erin Sweeney BS, is a Clinical Research Coordinator in the Department of Vascular Surgery at Massachusetts General Hospital, aiding in the facilitation of clinical trials for patients with PAD. Erin earned her Bachelor of Science degree from Villanova University in Psychology and Biology, graduating Cum Laude.

Contributors

Anahita Dua Vascular Surgery, Massachusetts General Hospital/ Harvard Medical School, Boston, MA, USA

Division of Vascular and Endovascular Surgery, Massachusetts General Hospital/Harvard Medical School, Boston, MA, USA

Lindsey Ferraro Vascular Surgery, Massachusetts General Hospital, Boston, MA, USA

Division of Vascular and Endovascular Surgery, Massachusetts General Hospital/Harvard Medical School, Boston, MA, USA

Gaurav Parmar Division of Vascular Medicine, Department of Cardiology, Massachusetts General Hospital/Harvard Medical School, Boston, MA, USA

Sara Rose-Sauld Podiatry, Massachusetts General Hospital, Boston, MA, USA

Nikolaos Zacharias Division of Vascular and Endovascular Surgery, Department of Surgery, Massachusetts General Hospital/ Harvard Medical School, Boston, MA, USA

Part I

Patient Identification

Selecting the Correct Patient Candidate

Anahita Dua, Sara Rose-Sauld, and Lindsey Ferraro

Patient selection for the TADV is fundamental to the success of the procedure. The ideal patient to undergo a TADV is one that has no other endovascular or open options for limb salvage. This is a patient with severe rest pain and a wound on the foot who has exhausted any other revascularization considerations *and* has small vessel disease of the foot. In a standard revascularization procedure, the clinician hopes to bridge the space between two acceptable flow targets either through open bypass or endovascular recanalization to achieve direct flow to the wound. However, in patients who are candidates for TADV distal targets in the arterial system are compromised or are of poor quality.

A. Dua (✉)
Vascular Surgery, Massachusetts General Hospital/Harvard Medical School, Boston, MA, USA
e-mail: ADUA1@mgh.harvard.edu

S. Rose-Sauld
Podiatry, Massachusetts General Hospital, Boston, MA, USA
e-mail: SROSE-SAULD@mgh.harvard.edu

L. Ferraro
Vascular Surgery, Massachusetts General Hospital, Boston, MA, USA
e-mail: LTFERRARO@mgh.harvard.edu

A. Dua et al. (eds.), *The Massachusetts General Hospital Approach to Transcatheter Arterialization of the Deep Veins for Advanced Limb Salvage*, https://doi.org/10.1007/978-3-031-37510-1_1

1.1   Profile of a TADV Patient

- More likely to be male (3:1 ratio M:F)
- Generally high levels of comorbidity, including:
  - Diabetes (more Type II than Type I)
  - HX smoking, hypertension, dyslipidemia
- Have a nonhealing ischemic wound present for many months
- Some present with contralateral amputation due to CLTI and are attempting to maintain the last bit of their mobility
- Two general pathways:
  - Well known to the system (prior revascularization attempts)
  - Amputation recommended by a nonspecialist as primary treatment

1.2   Major Considerations

- Critical considerations should include:
  - Uncontrolled infection
    - Osteomyelitis
      Abscess
  - Significant in-flow disease
  - Lack of viable donor vessel
  - **Patient compliance and support—this is a process, not just a procedure it will take commitment by the family, care team but most importantly the patient**
  - Subject history
  - Clinical snapshot
    - Ambulatory status, timeframe, and current state
        Bedridden; wheelchair; walking aids
        Walking without aid -> distances in meters
    - Activity level
    - Comorbidities that may affect the treatment or time-frame of wound healing, as well as survival to one year
    - Smoking
    - Dyslipidemia
    - Hypertension

- • Diabetes: years from diagnosis, Type I or II; neuropathy
- • Renal function: Creatinine <2.5 mg/dl.
- • Heart disease: LV dysfunction; CHF, Angina/MI; CABG/ PTCA; Afib; valvular disease
- – PAD etiology: Atherosclerosis; buerger/vasculitis; aneurysm; embolism; past surgical or interventional procedures on the current limb

Evaluating the Angiogram

2

Anahita Dua, Sara Rose-Sauld,
and Lindsey Ferraro

The first step in the TADV process after the identification of a potential patient is to objectively evaluate the angiogram. All patients that are being considered for the procedure should undergo a diagnostic angiogram that answers three questions: *(1) does the patient have inflow to the popliteal? (2) is there a remanent tibial vessel (ideally PT) that can be used as the proximal stent landing zone? (3) are there no other options for revascularization in this patient?* Using the "stoplight" approach in angiographic screening will help answer these key questions.

If the answer to all three of these questions is YES then this is a patient that may be ideal for TADV. At the MGH, we use a "stop light" approach to angiographic screening described below:

A. Dua (✉)
Vascular Surgery, Massachusetts General Hospital/Harvard Medical School, Boston, MA, USA
e-mail: ADUA1@mgh.harvard.edu

S. Rose-Sauld
Podiatry, Massachusetts General Hospital, Boston, MA, USA
e-mail: SROSE-SAULD@mgh.harvard.edu

L. Ferraro
Vascular Surgery, Massachusetts General Hospital, Boston, MA, USA
e-mail: LTFERRARO@mgh.harvard.edu

© The Author(s), under exclusive license to Springer Nature Switzerland AG 2023
A. Dua et al. (eds.), *The Massachusetts General Hospital Approach to Transcatheter Arterialization of the Deep Veins for Advanced Limb Salvage*, https://doi.org/10.1007/978-3-031-37510-1_2

2.1   Stoplight Approach to Angiographic Screening

- **Green—favorable (Figs. 2.1 and 2.2a)**
  - Access and inflow can accommodate a long interventional sheath. Large inflow vessels are relatively free from obstruction to place a 40+ cm sheath; calcium burden is low.
  - Very little to no inflow disease
- **Yellow—increased screening assessment, proceed with caution. (Fig. 2.2b)**
  - Access and inflow may accommodate a long interventional sheath. Possible with inflow treatment; calcium manageable with intervention.

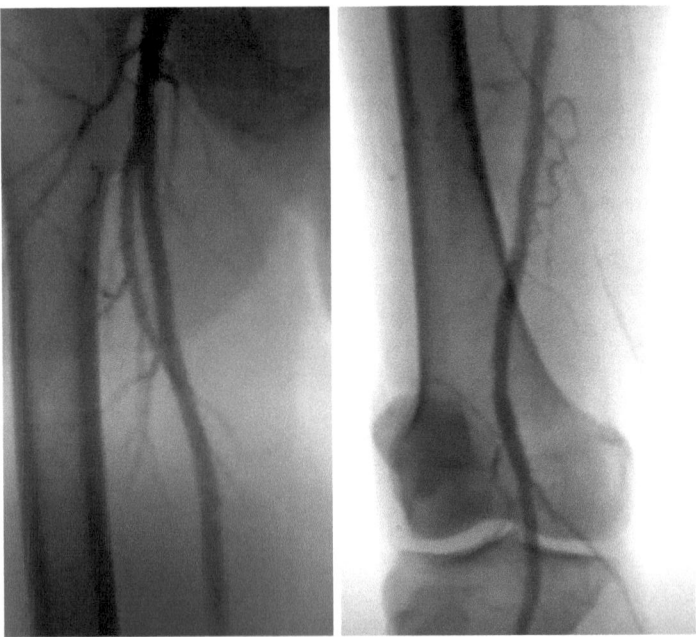

Fig. 2.1 Favorable angiogram showing large inflow vessels relatively free from obstruction

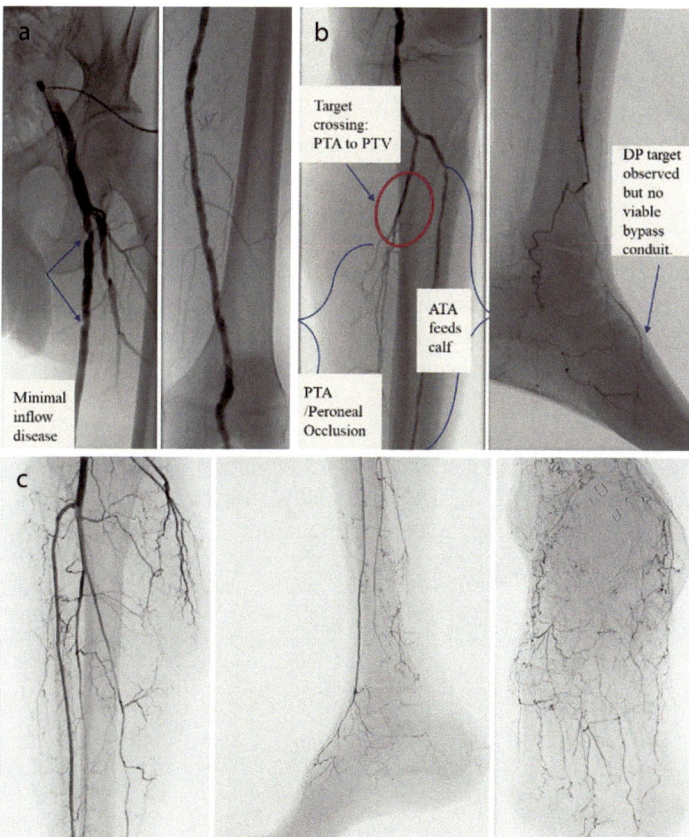

Fig. 2.2 Angiographic results showing (**a**) minimal inflow disease (green); (**b**) proceed with caution, separate inflow treatment may be needed; (**c**) not recommended to proceed with TADV, cannot accommodate a long sheath

- – **Moderate inflow disease should be possible to treat in the same setting. Consider how much time will be needed to treat inflow when deciding whether to stage and treat in a separate setting. (>1 h of work, treat separately)**
- • **Red—Not recommended. (Fig. 2.2c)**

– **Access and inflow cannot accommodate a long interventional sheath. Presence of long chronic total occlusion; highly visible untreated calcium burden.**
– **Long occlusions should be staged and treated prior to arterialization of the deep veins**

2.2   Tibial Donor Vessel Evaluation

- Once the full picture of the patient has been considered, assessing what the best donor artery (the vessel used to make the arteriovenous connection for the delivery of oxygenated blood to the foot) will be is key to success.
- *Ideal donor artery traits*:
    – Is not the main source of nutritive blood to the foot as time is needed for the TADV circuit to mature
    – There is at least a 2 cm landing zone for the tapered stent

Preprocedural Wound Considerations

3

Anahita Dua, Sara Rose-Sauld, and Lindsey Ferraro

Patients with non-healing wounds due to limited distal blood flow are ideal TADV candidates as the procedure will actively increase flow to the foot through arterialization of blood vessels. However, no amount of excellent blood flow will heal a wound if the patient does not have appropriate offloading and good infection control. Hence, the preprocedural evaluation and *optimization* of the wound are important. The goal post-procedure is to keep the wound as stable as possible (limit progression) giving the TADV a chance to mature before definitive wound care/procedures are undertaken. The WIfI classification system in conjunction with the stoplight approach will identify appropriate considerations for TADV and guide post-procedure wound care.

This chapter will detail the various presentations of wounds and the appropriate considerations for TADV.

A. Dua (✉)
Vascular Surgery, Massachusetts General Hospital/Harvard Medical School, Boston, MA, USA
e-mail: ADUA1@mgh.harvard.edu

S. Rose-Sauld
Podiatry, Massachusetts General Hospital, Boston, MA, USA
e-mail: SROSE-SAULD@mgh.harvard.edu

L. Ferraro
Vascular Surgery, Massachusetts General Hospital, Boston, MA, USA
e-mail: LTFERRARO@mgh.harvard.edu

© The Author(s), under exclusive license to Springer Nature Switzerland AG 2023
A. Dua et al. (eds.), *The Massachusetts General Hospital Approach to Transcatheter Arterialization of the Deep Veins for Advanced Limb Salvage*, https://doi.org/10.1007/978-3-031-37510-1_3

3.1 How to Identify Appropriate Wounds

What to look for:

- Wounds without uncontrolled infection
- Wounds that do not affect the lateral plantar vein even after minor amputation
- Wounds of the forefoot or superficial wounds of the mid and hindfoot
- Wounds stable enough to last the 4–6 weeks of TADV fistula maturation

The SVS WIfI [Wound (W), Ischemia (I) and foot Infection ("fI")] classification system for the threatened lower limb allows for a framework by which to gauge whether a foot with a wound is an appropriate candidate for TADV. The wound and foot infection components are of interest, as candidates have known Ischemia.

SVS Wound (W) Category

- Accounts for size, depth, severity, and complexity of healing. Grade 0 (rest pain) to 3 (deep ulcer ± calcaneal involvement ± extensive gangrene)

Wound Grade 1, An Appropriate Candidate (Fig. 3.1)
Small shallow ulcer; no exposed bone unless limited to the distal phalanx.

Wound Grade 2, Additional Considerations Required (Fig. 3.2)
Deeper ulcer with exposed bone, joint, or tendon, generally not involving the heel; shallow heel ulcer without calcaneal involvement.

X-ray or MRI to rule out osteomyelitis is recommended.

MRI/X-ray recommended to determine if appropriate for TADV.

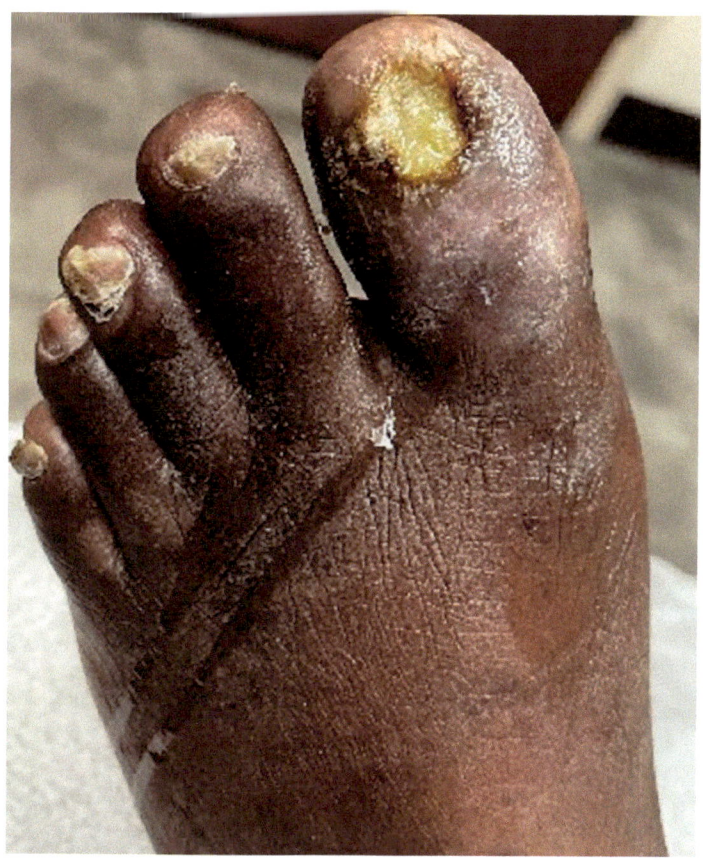

Fig. 3.1 An appropriate wound to proceed with TADV

Wound Grade 3, Additional Considerations Required (Fig. 3.3)

Extensive, deep ulcer involving forefoot and/or midfoot; deep, full-thickness heel ulcer with or without calcaneal involvement.

X-ray or MRI to rule out osteomyelitis. If osteomyelitis is present, TADV is not advisable.

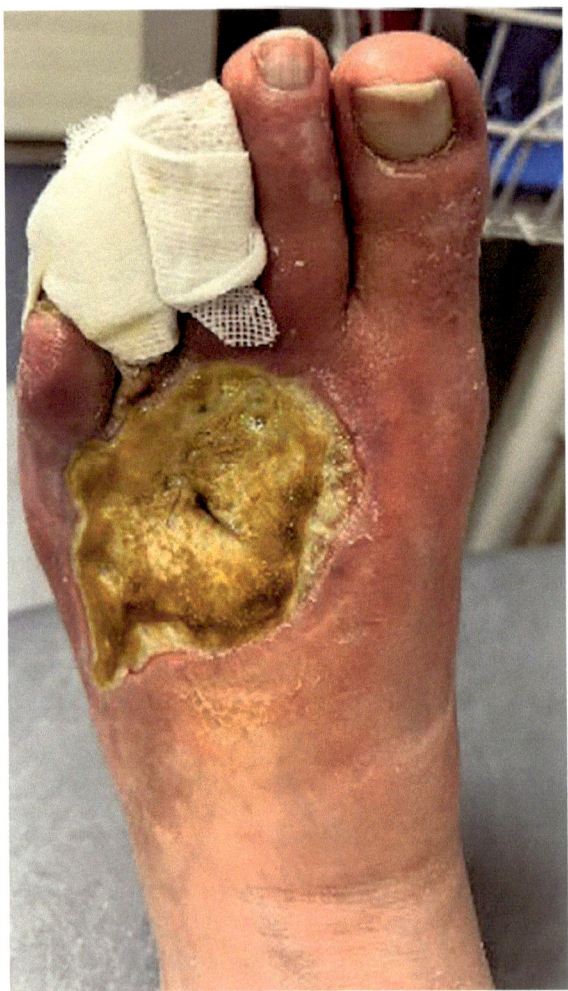

Fig. 3.2 Deep ulcer typically without heel involvement

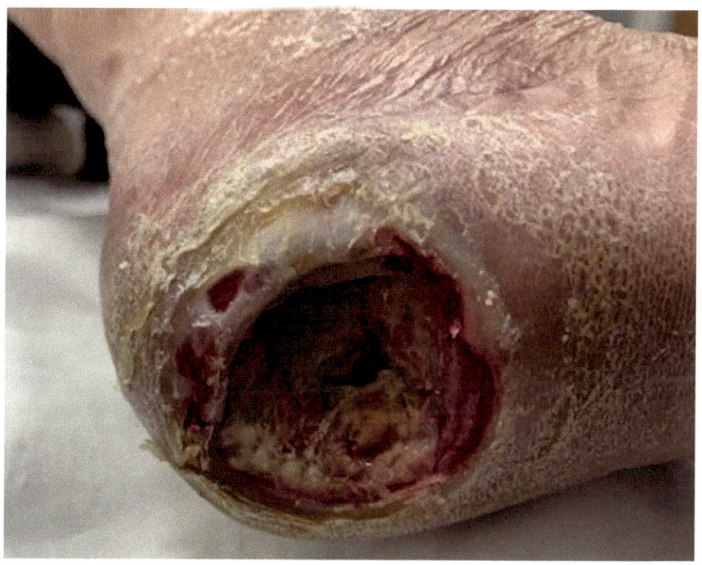

Fig. 3.3 Deep heel ulcer that requires MRI/X-ray to rule out osteomyelitis to determine if appropriate for TADV

SVS Foot Infection (fI) Category

Accounts for the presence and severity of infection.

Foot Infection Grade 0, An Appropriate Candidate (Fig. 3.4)

No symptoms or signs of infection or infection with local swelling or induration, erythema 0.5–2 cm around the ulcer, local tenderness or pain, local warmth, or purulent discharge.

Foot Infection Grade 1, An Appropriate Candidate (Fig. 3.5)

Local infection involving only the skin and the subcutaneous tissue <2 cm. Exclude other causes of inflammatory response of the skin (trauma, gout, acute Charcot, fracture, thrombosis, venous stasis).

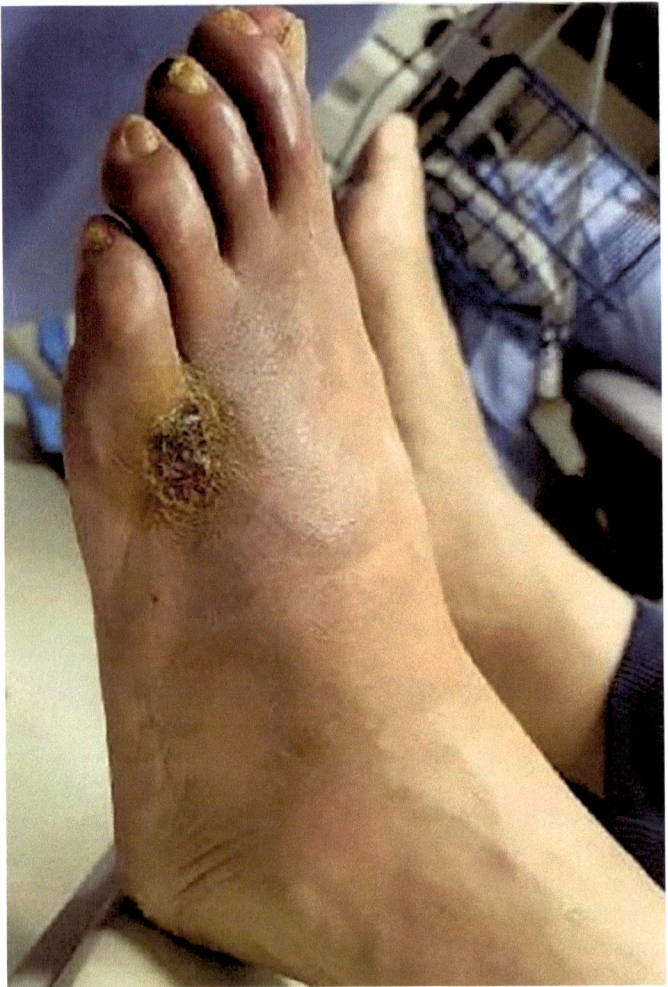

Fig. 3.4 No foot infection signs or symptoms seen. This is an appropriate candidate

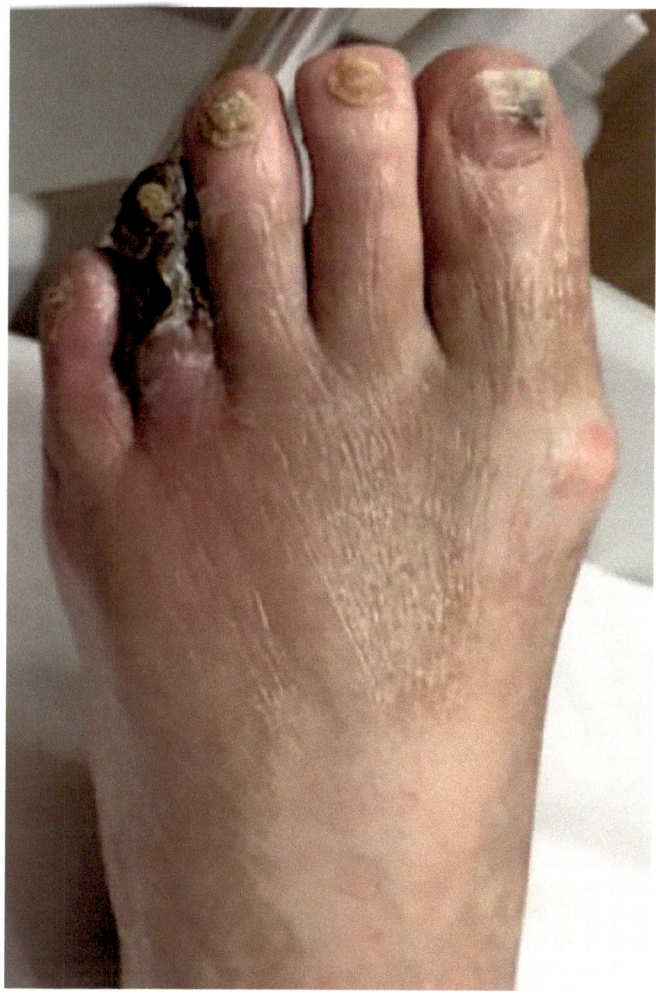

Fig. 3.5 Local infection of skin and subcutaneous tissue, this is an appropriate TADV candidate if local infection can be controlled

Foot Infection Grade 2, Additional Considerations Required (Fig. 3.6)

Local infection with erythema >2 cm, or involving structures deeper than skin and subcutaneous tissues.

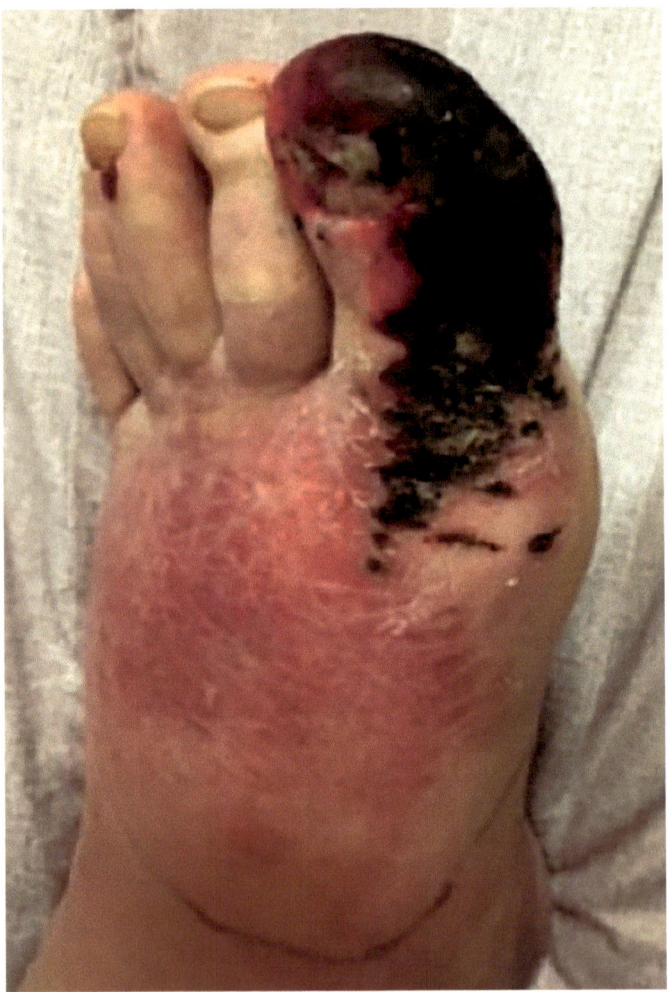

Fig. 3.6 Local infection with erythema >2 cm, or deeper than skin & subcutaneous level. Additional considerations required

Check blood infection markers and start with local antiseptics in combination with systemic antibiotics. Surgical debridement and/or minor amputation prior to TADV may be required. TADV procedure advisability is dependent upon infection control.

Foot Infection Grade 3, TADV Not Advisable (Fig. 3.7)

Local infection with Systemic Inflammatory Response Syndrome (SIRS).

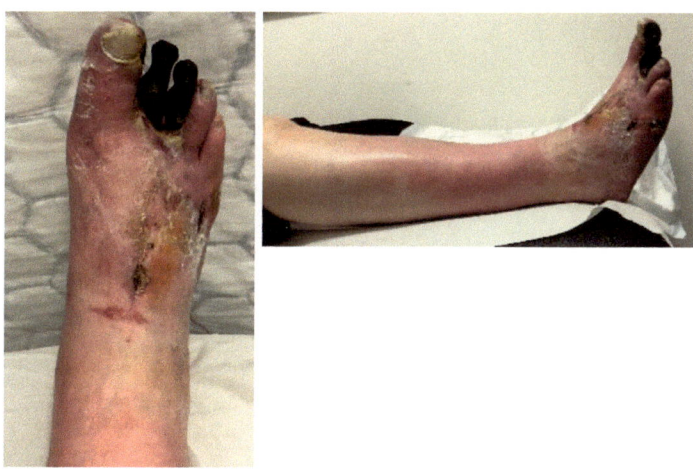

Fig. 3.7 Local infection with SIRS. This is not an appropriate TADV candidate

3.2   Stop Light Approach to Wound Screening, WIfI

- **Green—favorable** (Fig. 3.8)
  - **Wounds stable enough** to last the 4–6 weeks of fistula maturation
  - **Wounds that do not affect** the lateral plantar vein even after minor amputation

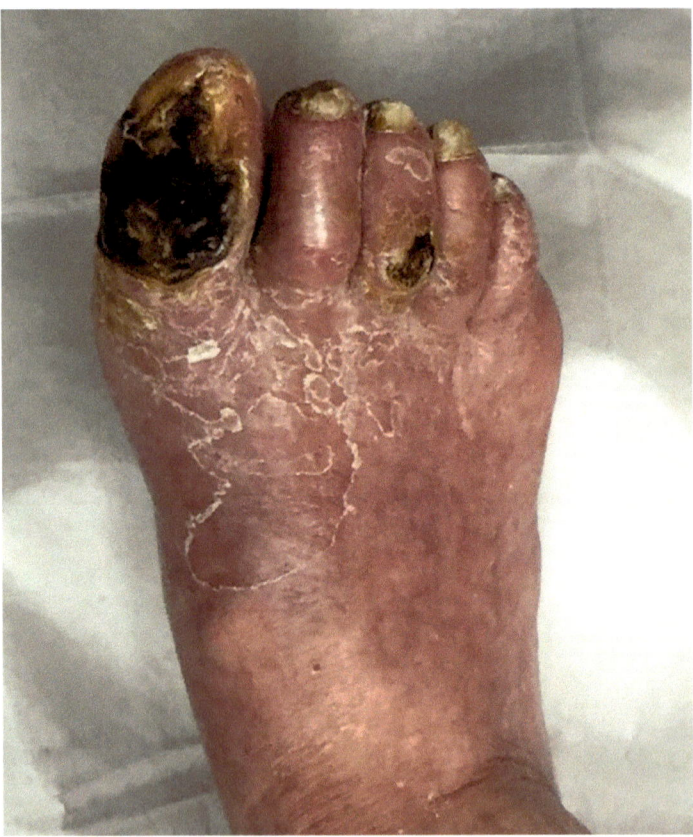

Fig. 3.8 Stable wound at the forefoot with no uncontrolled infection nor impact to the LPV

- **Wounds of the forefoot or superficial wounds** of the mid and hindfoot
- **Wounds without** uncontrolled infection
- **Yellow—increased screening assessment** (Fig. 3.9)
  - **Deep wounds with damage to deeper structures,** like exposed bones, tendons, and muscles (additional diagnostic needed)
  - X-ray, MRI
  - Wounds with clinical signs of local infection (additional diagnostic needed)
  - **Tissue biopsy, bone biopsy, blood marker**
  - **After evaluation of additional diagnostics, decide whether to proceed or not**

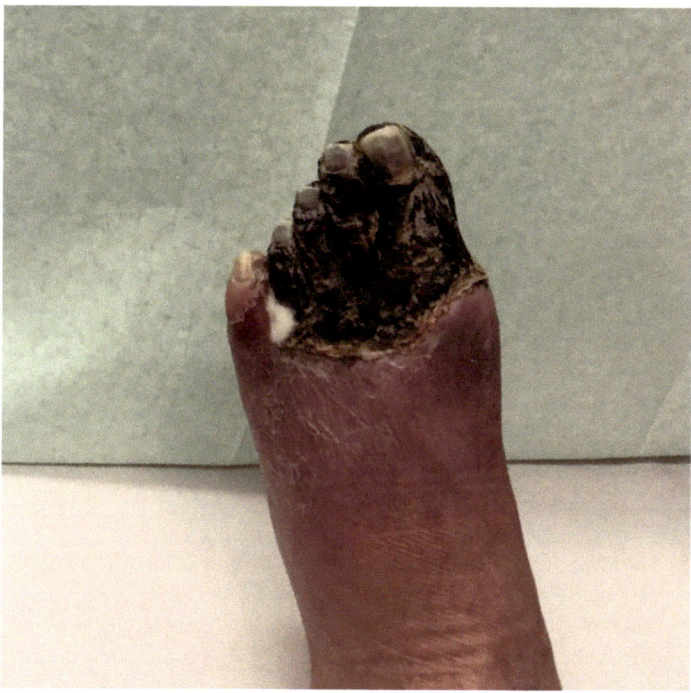

Fig. 3.9 Deep wounds damaging deeper structures or local infection, requiring additional diagnostics

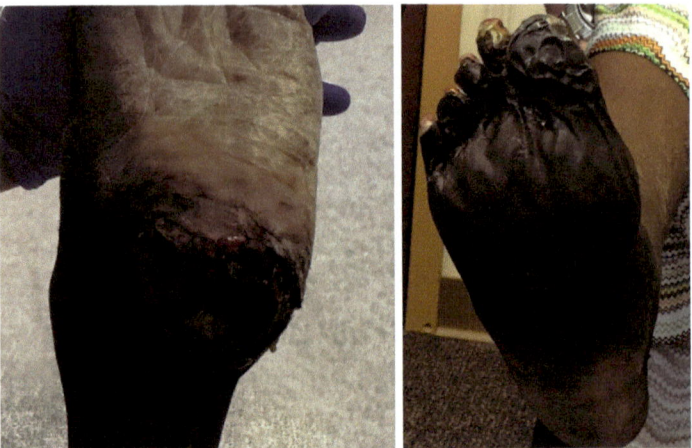

Fig. 3.10 Stop and assess risk/reward of TADV for patient that has wounds with demonstrable damage to deeper structures and infection

- **Red—stop—risk/reward for the patient assessed** (Fig. 3.10)
  - **Deep wounds with demonstrable damage** to deeper structures, like osteomyelitis, bone necrosis in the mid foot or rear foot.
  - *W - 3*
  - **Wounds with demonstrable clinical signs of infection,** local and systemic SIRS (**S**ystemic **I**nflammatory **R**esponse **S**yndrome)
  - *fI – 3*

3.3   Stop Light Approach to Wound Screening, Location (Fig. 3.11)

- **Green**—Involving the forefoot and little to no overlap with the metatarsal region.
- **Yellow**—Metatarsal region—assess how much tissue is salvageable.
- **Red**—Heel and/or ankle wound involvement. Risk/reward for limb and patient's ambulatory future.

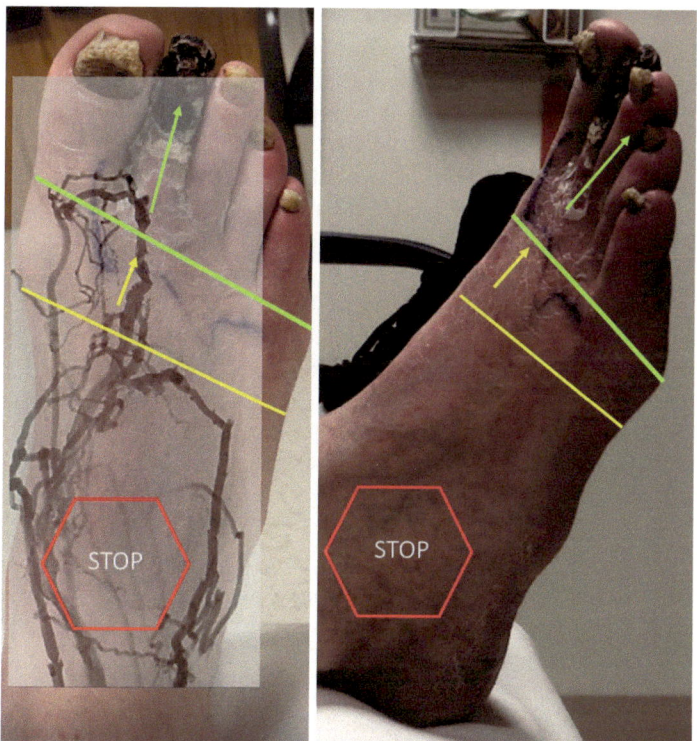

Fig. 3.11 Stoplight approach to wound screening, location

3.4   Pre-TADV Wound Stability

- The goal of wound care before TADV:
  - Maintain a dry, stable wound and control local infections.
  - Preserve as much tissue as possible
- Expectations:
  - Often some necrosis level occurs and will generally progress until the TADV is performed.
  - If there are wounds present, we do not expect to heal these wounds until at least 3 months after TADV. Plan to keep as stable as possible at this point, **rather than heal wounds.**

- **Given the longevity of wounds, close monitoring for infection and rapid treatment (surgical or non-surgical) are crucial for successful outcomes.**
- Surgery should be for source control of infections or excessive extension of necrotic tissue ONLY.
  - Resect infected soft tissue and bones (dry, necrotic tissue ok to leave) but wet gangrene, abscesses, and acute osteomyelitis must be resected. Repeat debridement until source control is obtained.
  - Large open wounds, exposed tendon, and bone OK if no local or systemic signs of infection arise (i.e., no leukocytosis, erythema, purulence, malodor, etc.)
- Daily wound care: Betadine-soaked gauze and dry dressings daily. Increase to BID if maceration occurs
  - No xeroform, no hydrogels. No compression
- Offload bilateral heels with pillows or offloading boots while in bed to prevent heel ulcers
  - If outpatient—weekly visits with wound care specialist along with home daily dressing changes.
  - If inpatient—a member of the wound care team performs dressing changes daily
- Weight-bearing status
  - Generally, if there is a plantar foot ulcer, non-weight bearing is necessary for total offloading
  - Consider touch-down weight bearing depending on the location and extent of the wound if the patient is physically capable
  - Consult physical therapy for assistance
    Knee scooters are often the preferred assistive device

Scenario #1

Wet Gangrene → resect infected, control ascending infection (Figs. 3.12 and 3.13)

- In this case admission, great toe amputation only, left open, close monitoring post-op
- Intra-op cultures to guide antibiotic management
- Infectious disease consult

Open amputation site- pack with wet to dry dressing.

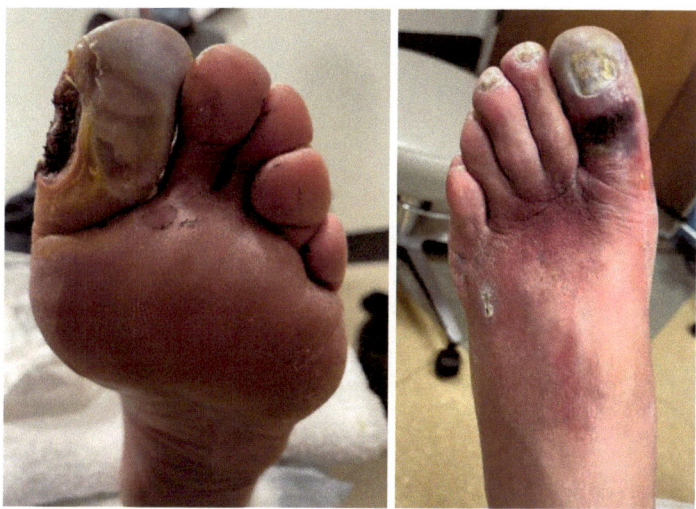

Fig. 3.12 Prior to great toe amputation

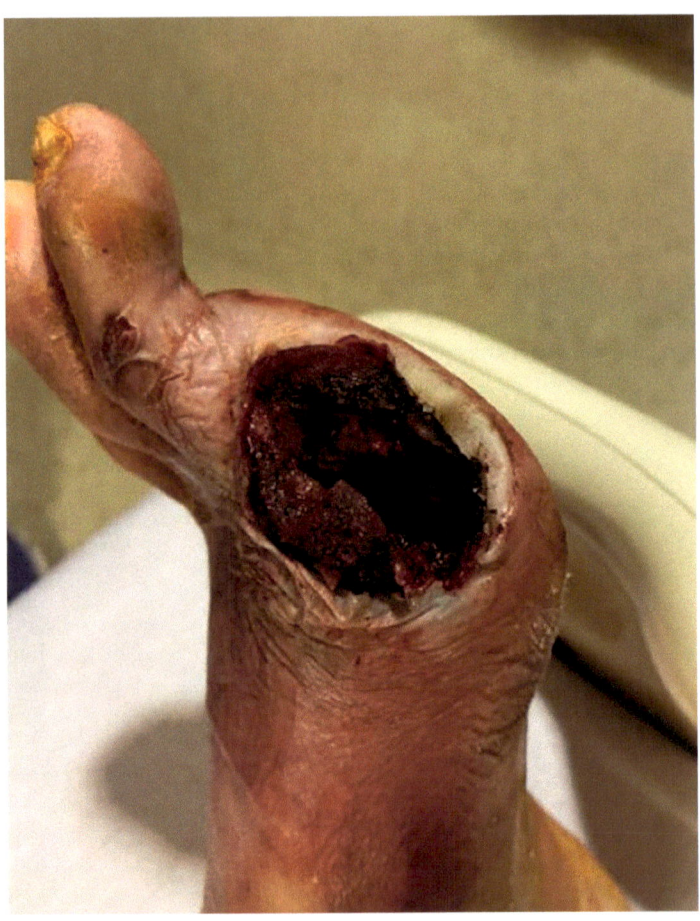

Fig. 3.13 Post-op great toe amputation

Scenario #2

Dry gangrene ➔ no surgery (Figs. 3.14 and 3.15)

- Betadine-soaked gauze and dry dressing daily

Scenario #3

Dry gangrene with some maceration ➔ betadine-soaked gauze twice daily and daily monitoring + non-weight-bearing (Figs. 3.16 and 3.17)

- If dries out after 2–7 days ➔ continue conservative management
- If erythema, malodor, or systemic signs of infection progress➔ debridement vs amputation, left open

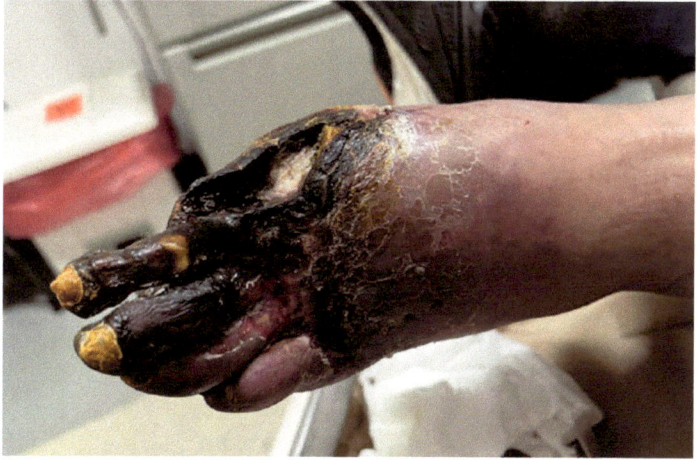

Fig. 3.14 Non-weight-bearing

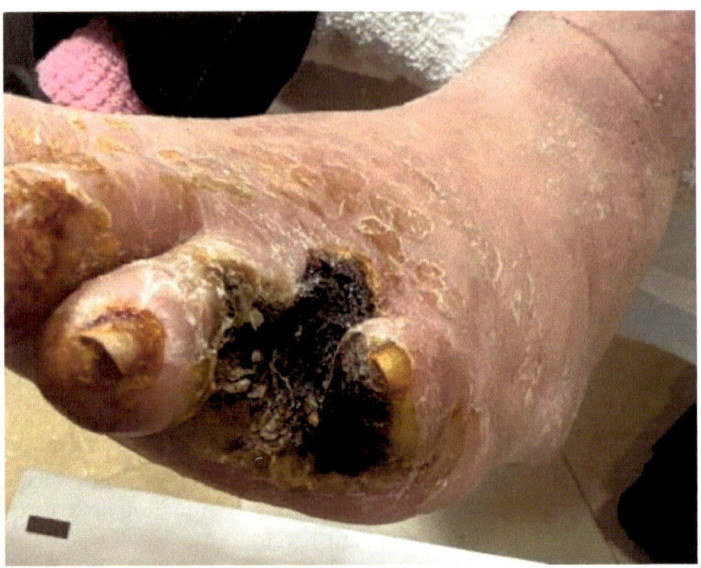

Fig. 3.15 Heel touch weight-bearing

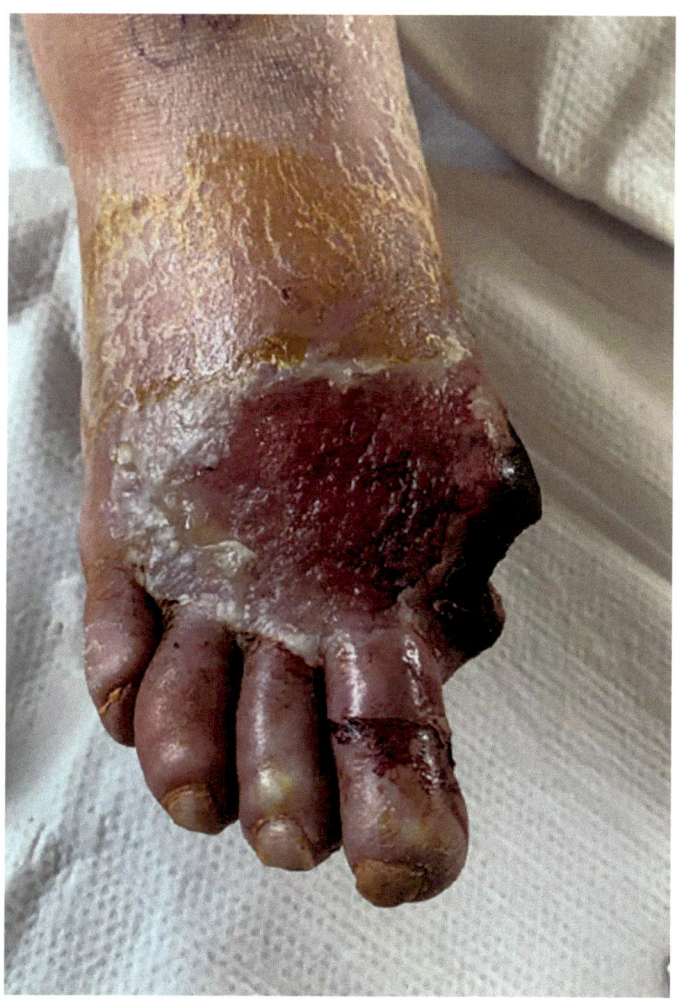

Fig. 3.16 Initial presentation

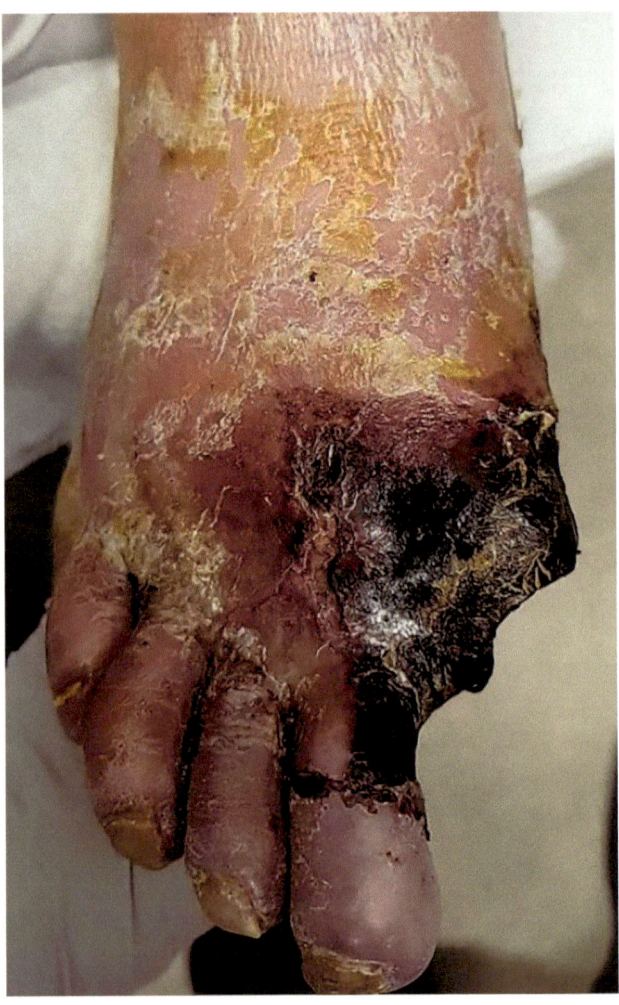

Fig. 3.17 7 days after modifying wound care

Explaining TADV to the Patient and Family

4

Anahita Dua, Sara Rose-Sauld,
and Lindsey Ferraro

A key factor to success is ensuring the patient and their family/support system are committed to the process of TADV, which is composed of three major stages. The expectations of the TADV procedure need to be discussed with the patient prior to moving forward. Some patients may experience swelling of the leg, pain in the foot requiring continuous narcotics, and worsening of wound requiring multiple admissions, antibiotics, persistent offloading, and debridement. Patients need to understand that even with TADV there is still a possibility of major amputation. It is imperative that the patient, support system, and medical team are educated and included in the care plan.

Managing expectations is the name of the game when discussing this procedure with patients. First and foremost, this is a limb salvage procedure and relies heavily on multidisciplinary commitment from both the members of the medical team and the

A. Dua (✉) · L. Ferraro
Division of Vascular and Endovascular Surgery, Massachusetts General Hospital/Harvard Medical School, Boston, MA, USA
e-mail: ADUA1@mgh.harvard.edu; LTFERRARO@mgh.harvard.edu

S. Rose-Sauld
Podiatry, Massachusetts General Hospital, Boston, MA, USA
e-mail: SROSE-SAULD@mgh.harvard.edu

patient/family. In discussion with the patient, we begin by explaining that TADV is not a magic bullet that will result in immediate blood flow to heal a wound, rather it is a process that has three major stages:

1. Is the patient a candidate for the procedure at all based on anatomy? (angiogram plus pedal mapping need to be completed to determine the answer)
2. Will the TADV flow be sufficient to arterialize the deep veins of the foot within 3 months and will the wound stay stable during this time?
3. Is the wound care and ultimate flow sufficient to heal the definitive procedure (typically a trans metatarsal amputation [TMA]) in 3 months?

Some patients will experience pain in the foot that requires persistent narcotics to manage in the time that the TADV is maturing as one does not want to rush into the removal of the necrotic tissue. Some patients will have severe swelling of the leg although this is less than in open, surgical DVA procedures. Some patients will have worsening of their wounds that require multiple admissions for debridement, a PICC line with antibiotics, and persistent offloading such that they may need a rehabilitation facility. As a result, given the major lift on the part of the patient, one of the crucial elements of success is patient and family commitment. The following points should be addressed and agreed upon during the consultation before agreeing to provide the procedure:

- Patient support is an important part of the TADV process. (Spouse, Adult Children, Friend, Professional Services)
- The patient understands that pain, swelling, multiple procedures, multiple ultrasound evaluations, and likely offloading (non-weight-bearing) may occur for up to 12 months postprocedure
- Patient understands that even with TADV there is a possibility of a major amputation (above or below knee)

- All the key caregivers identified, trained, and included in the care plan

IF THE PATIENT IS IN AGREEMENT, THE FAMILY IS IN AGREEMENT AND THE CARE TEAM IS IN AGREEMENT, IT IS TIME TO PREPARE THE PATIENT FOR TADV.

Part II

Patient Preparation

Duplex Pedal Mapping for Case Preparation

5

Anahita Dua, Sara Rose-Sauld, and Lindsey Ferraro

5.1 Introduction

Prior to undergoing TADV, a duplex pedal mapping ultrasound is necessary to evaluate the lower extremity deep venous and arterial system for the presence of deep vein thrombosis and adequate venous size for use of TADV and to evaluate the arterial flow to the foot. The evaluation includes a limited lower extremity venous duplex evaluation to rule out thrombus of the popliteal, posterior tibial, and peroneal veins as well as to assess initial (pre-op) arterial flow to the foot via the distal posterior tibial, distal peroneal, and distal anterior tibial arteries at the level of the ankle. Additionally, diameter measurements (AP & Transverse) are obtained for the great saphenous vein, the posterior tibial veins, the medial marginal vein, and the lateral plantar vein. This comprehensive evaluation will ensure that patients are optimally prepared for TADV.

A. Dua (✉) · L. Ferraro
Division of Vascular and Endovascular Surgery, Massachusetts General Hospital/Harvard Medical School, Boston, MA, USA
e-mail: ADUA1@mgh.harvard.edu; LTFERRARO@mgh.harvard.edu

S. Rose-Sauld
Podiatry, Massachusetts General Hospital, Boston, MA, USA
e-mail: SROSE-SAULD@mgh.harvard.edu

© The Author(s), under exclusive license to Springer Nature Switzerland AG 2023
A. Dua et al. (eds.), *The Massachusetts General Hospital Approach to Transcatheter Arterialization of the Deep Veins for Advanced Limb Salvage*, https://doi.org/10.1007/978-3-031-37510-1_5

Purpose

To evaluate the lower extremity deep venous and arterial system for the presence of deep vein thrombosis and adequate venous size for use of TADV and to evaluate the arterial flow to the foot.

Indications and Limitations

(a) Pre-operative evaluation for TADV placement.
(b) Presence of open wounds, burns, casts, or surgical dressings.
(c) Inability of patient to cooperate for exam.

Equipment

(a) Duplex imaging equipment with linear 7–9 MHz and/or linear 8–18i MHz (hockey stick probe).

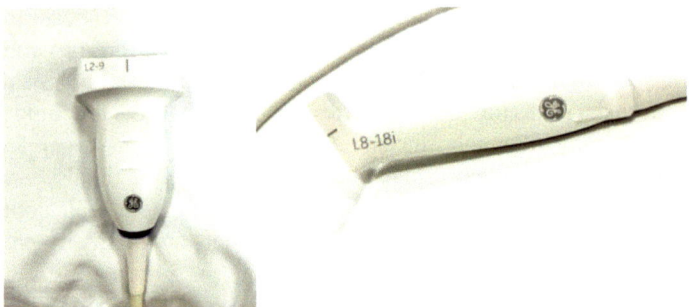

(b) PACS (Picture Archiving and Communications System).
(c) Acoustic coupling gel.
(d) Towels/washcloths.

Patient Prep

(a) Introduction to the patient, verification of patient information, and a brief explanation of what the exam will entail.

(b) Obtain any pertinent patient history.
(c) Have the patient remove any pants, socks, and shoes.
(d) Position the patient in the supine position on the table, drape the patient to maintain privacy, and unwrap any dressings that may be present on the patient.
(e) Once the patient's foot is unwrapped, have the patient externally rotate their leg on the exam table that is in a reverse Trendelenburg position.

Procedure

(a) Evaluation for deep vein thrombosis of the lower extremity
- Equipment gain and display settings should be optimized to provide the best grayscale images. Color duplex is utilized to assist in identifying vessels and flow disturbances.
- A limited lower extremity venous duplex evaluation must be done to rule out thrombus of the popliteal, posterior tibial, and peroneal veins.
- Begin by placing the transducer at the level of the popliteal fossa.
- In a transverse projection, the popliteal vein is identified and intermittent compressions are performed.
- Pulse wave Doppler is then used in a longitudinal plane to evaluate the vein for spontaneous flow, respiratory variation, and/or flow augmentation.
- The posterior tibial and peroneal veins are evaluated in the transverse plane from the level of the distal popliteal fossa to the medial malleolus documenting evidence of compressibility and augmentation with color.
(b) Evaluation of the lower extremity arterial exam
- Equipment gain and display settings should be optimized to provide the best possible grayscale images. Color duplex is utilized to assist in identifying vessels and flow disturbances.
- A limited lower extremity arterial duplex evaluation must be done to evaluate initial (pre-op) arterial flow to the foot

via the distal posterior tibial, distal peroneal, and distal anterior tibial arteries at the level of the ankle.

- Begin by placing the transducer at the level of the ankle.
- The arteries are evaluated in longitudinal view with gray-scale and/or color duplex and spectral pulse wave Doppler.
- Pulse wave Doppler must be obtained in the longitudinal plane at an angle of ≤60 degrees, keeping the cursor aligned parallel with the flow.

(c) Evaluation of the lower extremity veins for mapping

- Equipment gain and display settings should be optimized to provide the best possible grayscale images. Color duplex is utilized to assist in identifying vessels and flow disturbances.
- The great saphenous vein is evaluated in the transverse plane at the level of the ankle. Diameter measurements (AP & Transverse) are obtained.
- The posterior tibial veins are evaluated in the transverse plane at the level of the medial malleolus. Diameter measurements (AP & Transverse) are obtained.
- The medial marginal vein is evaluated in the transverse plane at the level of the proximal to distal dorsal foot. Diameter measurements (AP & Transverse) are obtained.

The Medial Marginal Vein is located on the dorsum aspect of the foot - it is a continuation of the Dorsal venous arch of the foot and is the origin of the Great Saphenous Vein (it can be followed from the great saphenous vein to along the top of the arch of the foot towards the great toe).

- The lateral plantar vein is evaluated in the transverse plane at the level of the proximal to distal foot. Diameter measurements (AP & Transverse) are obtained.

The Lateral Plantar Vein is located along the plantar aspect of the foot and gives rise to the posterior tibial veins (it can be followed from the posterior tibial veins onto the plantar aspect of the foot and will move laterally fairly quickly).

5.2   Required Documentation

All images are stored on PACS.

Venous

(a) Dual screen grayscale images with and without transverse transducer compression are recorded for the following:
- Popliteal vein
- Posterior tibial veins
- Peroneal veins

(b) Spectral Doppler waveforms showing phasicity and augmentation are performed and recorded for the popliteal vein.

(c) Color duplex is used to further document flow in any segment of the deep venous system.

Arterial

(d) Long-axis grayscale images and/or color Doppler images must be documented and include the following:
- Distal posterior tibial artery at the ankle
- Distal peroneal artery at the ankle
- Distal anterior tibial artery at the ankle (Fig. 5.1).

Mapping

(a) Diameter measurements (AP & Transverse) of the veins are recorded at the following levels:

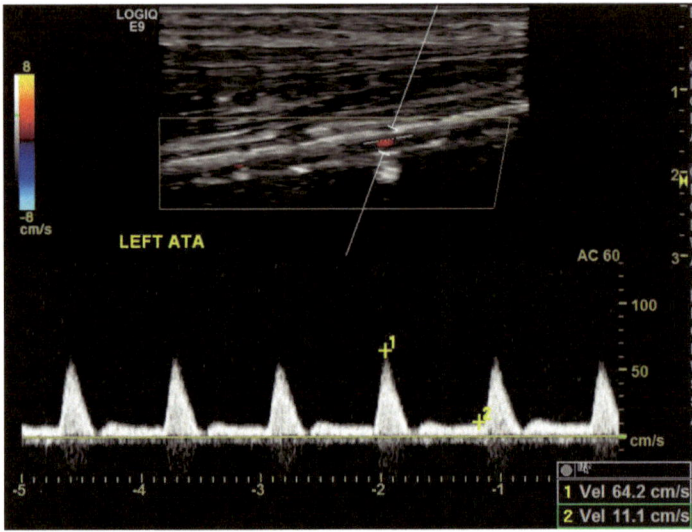

Fig. 5.1 Anterior tibial artery pre-op evaluation

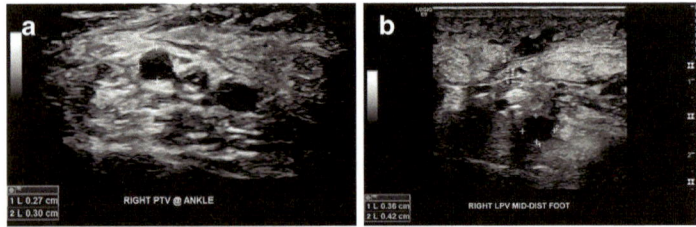

Fig. 5.2 (**a**) Pre-op mapping; (**b**) Pre-op mapping

- Posterior tibial veins at medial malleolus (Fig. 5.2a)
- Greater saphenous vein at the ankle
- Medial marginal vein (dorsal)
  - Proximal foot
  - Mid foot
  - Distal foot
- Lateral plantar vein (plantar) (Fig. 5.2b)

 – Proximal foot
 – Mid foot
 – Distal foot

5.3   Interpretation

Venous

(a) Normal exam (Fig. 5.3)
   • Spectral Doppler waveforms will demonstrate phasicity, spontaneity, and/or adequate augmentation.
   • Grayscale imaging will demonstrate the compressibility of all vessels and no evidence of echogenic material within the lumen.
(b) Abnormal exam (Fig. 5.4)
   • Spectral Doppler waveforms will demonstrate abnormal waveforms (absence of flow, continuous flow, etc. depending on the level of acuity).
   • Grayscale imaging will demonstrate incompressibility and dilation of the vein (again depending on the acuity).

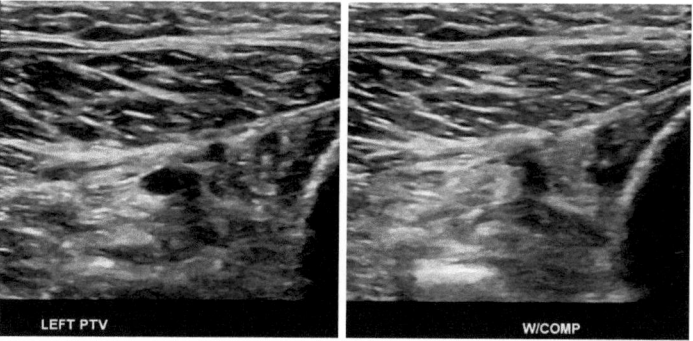

Fig. 5.3 PTV with compression—normal venous exam

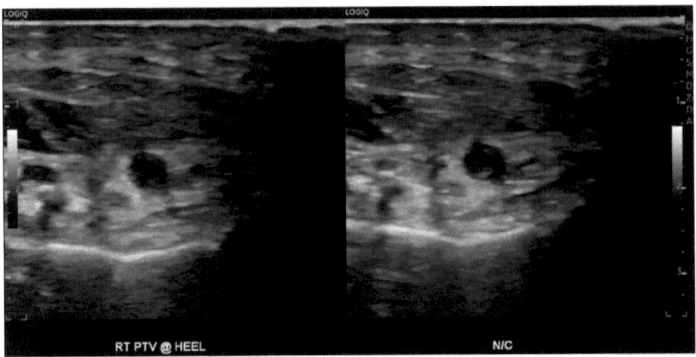

Fig. 5.4 PTV non-compressible—abnormal venous exam

Mapping

(a) Normal: A vein diameter of ≥3.0 mm is considered adequate size as well as compressibility (no thrombus or mural thickening).
(b) Abnormal: Vein diameters of ≤3.0 mm and/or thrombus/thick walls are considered inadequate.

Preoperative Optimization of the Patient

6

Anahita Dua, Gaurav Parmar,
Sara Rose-Sauld, and Lindsey Ferraro

Preoperative optimization of TADV patients revolves around three key areas: patient history, a physical exam, and optimizing medical conditions. Patients should be advised on exercise, diet, and smoking cessation prior to the TADV procedure. In addition, the care team must focus on optimizing medical conditions such as coronary artery disease, chronic kidney disease, hypertension, diabetes, and dyslipidemia by obtaining up-to-date preoperative lab values, physiologic testing, and imaging. Clinicians must take into consideration a patient's current anticoagulation therapy and determine the most appropriate antithrombotic therapy to be used preoperatively. Proper control of these factors will help promote a successful TADV outcome.

A. Dua
Vascular Surgery, Massachusetts General Hospital/Harvard Medical School, Boston, MA, USA
e-mail: ADUA1@mgh.harvard.edu

G. Parmar (✉)
Vascular Medicine Section, Division of Cardiology, Massachusetts General Hospital, Boston, MA, USA
e-mail: gmparmar@mgh.harvard.edu

S. Rose-Sauld
Podiatry, Massachusetts General Hospital, Boston, MA, USA
e-mail: SROSE-SAULD@mgh.harvard.edu

L. Ferraro
Vascular Surgery, Massachusetts General Hospital, Boston, MA, USA
e-mail: LTFERRARO@mgh.harvard.edu

© The Author(s), under exclusive license to Springer Nature Switzerland AG 2023
A. Dua et al. (eds.), *The Massachusetts General Hospital Approach to Transcatheter Arterialization of the Deep Veins for Advanced Limb Salvage*, https://doi.org/10.1007/978-3-031-37510-1_6

45

6.1   History

- A detailed history of leg symptoms, systemic risk factors, cardiovascular, and other comorbidities.
- Identify other conditions which can mimic symptoms of claudication and ischemic rest pain.
- Identify other etiologies of leg ulcers that may require different treatment approaches.
- The Wound, Ischemia, and foot Infection (WIfI) scoring system should be used to stage the Chronic Limb-Threatening Ischemia (CLTI) lesion/wound and to assess the need for revascularization. Alternatively, the Global Limb Anatomical Staging System (GLASS) can be considered.
- It is important to discuss and establish the goals of the procedure.
- Smoking
    - Tobacco cessation is essential before any interventional treatment for CLTI.
    - A multidisciplinary multimodal comprehensive approach is necessary for successful tobacco cessation.
    - All adults should be assessed at every healthcare visit for tobacco use.
    - To achieve tobacco abstinence, all adults who use tobacco should be firmly advised to quit.
    - A combination of behavioral interventions plus pharmacotherapy is recommended to maximize quit rates.
    - To facilitate tobacco cessation, it is reasonable to dedicate trained staff to tobacco cessation treatment team in every healthcare system
- Diet.
    - A diet emphasizing the intake of vegetables, fruits, legumes, nuts, whole grains, and fish is recommended.
    - Replacement of saturated fat with dietary monounsaturated and polyunsaturated fats should be encouraged.
    - A diet containing reduced amounts of cholesterol and sodium can be beneficial.

- As a part of a healthy diet, it is reasonable to minimize the intake of processed meat, refined carbohydrates, and sweetened beverages.
- As a part of a healthy diet, the intake of trans fats should be avoided.
- Exercise
  - Supervised exercise therapy should be considered if the patient can perform it, especially if claudication symptoms are present.
  - If a supervised regimen isn't available, home-based or upper extremity-based activity should be recommended to improve cardiovascular conditioning.
  - Adults should be routinely counseled in healthcare visits to optimize a physically active lifestyle.
  - Adults should engage in at least 150 minutes per week of accumulated moderate-intensity or 75 minutes per week of vigorous-intensity aerobic physical activity (or an equivalent combination of moderate and vigorous activity).
  - For adults unable to meet the minimum physical activity recommendations (at least 150 minutes per week of accumulated moderate-intensity or 75 minutes per week of vigorous-intensity aerobic physical activity), engaging in some moderate- or vigorous-intensity physical activity, even if less than this recommended amount, can be beneficial.
  - Decreasing sedentary behavior in adults should be recommended.

6.2   Physical Examination

- A detailed physical exam is always required before any procedure.
- The presence of S3 or elevated jugular venous pressure (JVP) may help understand the status of heart function/failure.
- Murmurs may indicate underlying valvular abnormalities.
- Carotid bruit suggests higher generalized atherosclerotic burden.

- Peripheral pulses should be examined to help understand the atherosclerotic involvement of the arteries of the extremities.
- The presence of peripheral/pedal edema may point toward a mixed-etiology (arterial and venous) ulcer, which may also require treatment for chronic venous insufficiency.

6.3 Optimizing Medical Conditions

- Coronary Artery Disease (CAD)
  - Advanced testing, such as an echocardiogram or cardiac catheterization, is generally neither required nor suggested unless the patient is symptomatic.
  - It is reasonable to obtain an electrocardiogram (ECG) pre-procedurally as it may unmask underlying CAD
- Chronic kidney disease (CKD)
  - Close monitoring of renal functions in patients with CKD is essential.
  - Avoiding nephrotoxic agents such as non-steroidal anti-inflammatory drugs (NSAID), angiotensin-converting enzyme inhibitors (ACEI), and angiotensin receptor blockers (ARB) immediately before TADV is a reasonable strategy.
- Hypertension
  - The goal is to maintain blood pressure at a reasonable level and not allow it to climb very high (Avoid BP > 180/100).
  - However, avoid hypotension as it may increase the risk of conduit thrombosis and may lead to failure of the TADV.
  - There is no data-driven preference in the choice of antihypertensive agent. However, ACEI or ARB provide overall benefits in cardiovascular outcomes as long as the renal function is normal. They should not be instituted in the immediate preprocedural period.
- Diabetes
  - Optimizing blood sugar is essential for diabetic patients.
  - The goal hemoglobin a1c is <7.
  - Avoid overt hypoglycemia.

- Long-acting insulin is generally avoided in the immediate preprocedural period.
- There is some evidence to suggest that Metformin, SGLT2i (sodium/glucose cotransporter-2 inhibitors), and GLP (glucagon-like peptide-1) agonists provide some benefits in limb-related outcomes in CLTI patients.
- It is reasonable to avoid canagliflozin in patients with prior history of amputation. The initial association has not been reproducible, and there is no definitive proof that class effect exists for SGLT2i.
- Dyslipidemia.
    - Target LDL is <70 and <55 if polyvascular disease is present.
    - Some studies and experts believe in a lower LDL target (<40).
    - Statin therapy should be initiated if not already started.
    - Statin therapy should be initiated irrespective of LDL level as it has been shown to improve life and limb outcomes due to its anti-inflammatory and pleiotropic effects.
    - If LDL is not at goal, then add ezetimibe to the statin therapy.
    - PCSK9i (proprotein convertase subtilisin/kexin type 9 inhibitor) should be considered in patients with familial hypercholesterolemia or with LDL not at goal despite being on statin therapy or ezetimibe.

6.4   Investigations

- Laboratory testing
    - Obtain complete blood count (CBC), chemistry profile, renal functions, liver functions, and coagulation profile (PT/INR).
    - If not available recently, then also obtain hemoglobin a1c and lipid panel for appropriate risk stratification.
- Physiologic testing
    - It is prudent to have the ankle-brachial pressure index (ABI), toe pressures, toe-brachial pressure index (TBI), and peripheral pulse volume recordings (PVRs) preoperatively.

- Apart from diagnosis, it also helps with a new baseline and for the follow-up to compare post-TADV (deep venous arterialization).
- Imaging
  - Axial imaging such as computerized tomographic angiogram (CTA), magnetic resonance imaging angiogram (MRA), or catheter-based angiography should be considered for procedure planning but not required for routine screening.

6.5   Antithrombotic Therapy

- Antithrombotic therapy
  - Antiplatelet therapy should be instituted with aspirin or clopidogrel or a combination of aspirin and clopidogrel, depending on the presence of other cardiovascular diseases.
  - Anticoagulation therapy is not indicated in the absence of polyvascular disease preoperatively.
  - Triple therapy with dual-antiplatelet therapy (DAPT) and an oral factor-Xa inhibitor is preferred, especially if the stenting is employed and an endovascular approach is utilized for TADV. Otherwise, DPI (Dual Pathway Inhibition) with a combination of antiplatelet monotherapy and an oral factor-Xa inhibitor should be instituted after the procedure.
  - For chronically anticoagulated patients, anticoagulation therapy should be discontinued preoperatively to minimize bleeding complications.
    Warfarin should be discontinued 4–5 days in advance.
    Oral factor-Xa inhibitor should be held for 48–72 hours before TADV.
    The decision of bridging with parenteral unfractionated heparin (UFH) can be considered on a case-by-case basis depending on the primary indication for the anticoagulation and thrombosis risk.

Part III

Procedure and Acute Post-operative Care

Overview of TADV and Required Equipment

7

Anahita Dua, Sara Rose-Sauld, and Lindsey Ferraro

Performing the TADV procedure requires skill and adequate materials. TADV can be done off the shelf with endovascular materials readily available but at the MGH we utilize the LimFlow System. In the chapter, we have detailed our approach but in areas where the LimFlow system is not available, we have detailed alternatives that can be used off the shelf. The ancillary devices required for a successful TADV procedure are outlined in conjunction with anatomical considerations that may impact the procedure.

7.1 Anatomical Considerations

Procedure length impacted by anatomical and comorbidity variability (Table 7.1):

A. Dua (✉) · L. Ferraro
Division of Vascular and Endovascular Surgery, Massachusetts General Hospital/Harvard Medical School, Boston, MA, USA
e-mail: ADUA1@mgh.harvard.edu; LTFERRARO@mgh.harvard.edu

S. Rose-Sauld
Podiatry, Massachusetts General Hospital, Boston, MA, USA
e-mail: SROSE-SAULD@mgh.harvard.edu

Table 7.1 Procedure length impacted by anatomical and comorbidity variability

Variable	Complexity-impact on procedure
Body habitus and arterial disease	Access and closure difficulty increases with larger habitus and disease presence in the access location
Arterial disease progression	Heavy calcification requires additional treatment and increases the difficulty in manipulating catheters within the arterial circuit
Prior implants in the circuit	Extra care and time are needed to manipulate through existing implants in the arterial system
Venous variability	Venous tortuosity, caliber, and presence of venous disease increase the time needed to successfully traverse and create the new arterialized circuit
Wound status and prior intervention	Pedal access may be prolonged due to extensive edema or the presence of a wound on the plantar surface

7.2 Equipment

- Ancillary devices
  - Access sheath
    4F Pedal MicroAccess Kit (Cook recommended)
    4/5F slender sheath (Terumo recommended)
    7F long (40+ cm) sheath (Terumo Destination recommended)
  - Sterile Esmarch or sterile pneumatic cuff
  - Several specialty guidewires (300 cm length)
    0.018″ AND 0.014″
    IFU-conform Crossing Wire (e.g. Medtronic NITREX, Terumo Runthrough, Boston Scientific Thruway)
  - Angiographic ruler (LeMaitre or CSI)
  - Guiding catheters (NaviCross or CXI)
    0.035″ and/or 0.18″ (minimal angle or straight)
    Long shaft (for navigation or wire exchange)

- PTA balloons
  0.018″ AND 0.014″
  Long shaft
  Diameters from 2.5 to 6.0 in various lengths of 40–200 mm
- LimFlow product kit
  - ARC arterial device (alternative: outback re-entry Cordis crossing catheter)
  - V-CEIVER venous snaring device (alternative: 5 mm × 150 mm POBA). Merit multi loop snare as well (ENSnare)
  - VECTOR antegrade valvulotome (alternative: 5 mm × 150 mm POBA to disrupt values)
  - LimFlow STENTs extension stents and crossing (tapered) stent (alternative: Viabahn 5 mm stent [Gore])
- Potential extra use
  - High pressure or cutting balloon in 5 and/or 6 mm long shaft (for residual valves around the ankle—25% of the cases)
  - DEB and/or DES in 3.5 or 4.0 mm
    Embolization coils 5.0–10.0 mm (knock out outflow veins to optimize flow—5% of cases at baseline).

Pedal Venous Access

8

Anahita Dua, Sara Rose-Sauld,
and Lindsey Ferraro

Achieving pedal venous access requires adequate preparation and knowledge of both the dorsal and plantar venous anatomy, emphasizing the lateral plantar vein as the primary access point. To ensure optimal outcomes, conducting a preoperative pedal venous ultrasound to assess diameter measurements, compressibility, and patency of the Lateral Plantar Veins (LPV) is necessary. It is crucial to characterize the tortuosity, pathology, and/or prominent valves of the LPV in addition to marking access points as distal as possible of the dominant LPV for a smooth execution of gaining pedal venous access. An optional, but recommended, step includes mapping and marking the pedal dorsal veins for potential access points. During the pedal venous ultrasound, it is important to note the presence of any thrombosed or absent pedal veins.

A. Dua (✉) · L. Ferraro
Division of Vascular and Endovascular Surgery, Massachusetts General Hospital/Harvard Medical School, Boston, MA, USA
e-mail: ADUA1@mgh.harvard.edu; LTFERRARO@mgh.harvard.edu

S. Rose-Sauld
Podiatry, Massachusetts General Hospital, Boston, MA, USA
e-mail: SROSE-SAULD@mgh.harvard.edu

8.1   Required Knowledge Base

- Dorsal venous anatomy
  - Dorsal venous arch
  - Medial marginal—can be used for diagnostic venograms
  - Greater saphenous
  - Anterior tibial
- Plantar venous anatomy
  - Lateral plantar—primary access point
  - Medial plantar
  - Posterior tibial
  - Lateral marginal

8.2   Preoperative Pedal Venous Ultrasound

- Pedal dorsal veins (Fig. 8.1)
  - Assess patency and diameter (AP) of the greater saphenous at the ankle to the medial marginal on the dorsal foot
  - Optional—map and mark veins for potential access points
- Pedal plantar veins (Fig. 8.1)
  - Confirm compressibility and patency of Lateral Plantar Veins (LPV) on the plantar aspect of the foot
  - Obtain diameter measurements of the dominant PTV at the ankle, LPV at the proximal foot, and LPV at the mid-distal

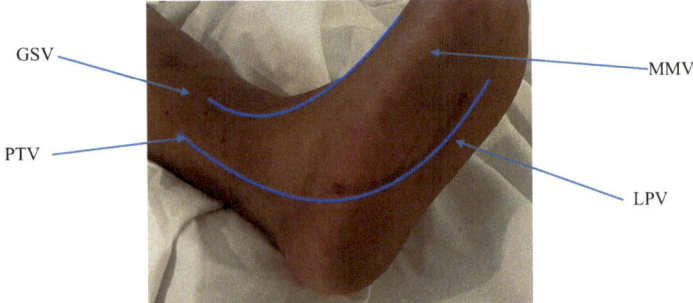

Fig. 8.1 Pedal dorsal and plantar veins for preoperative examination

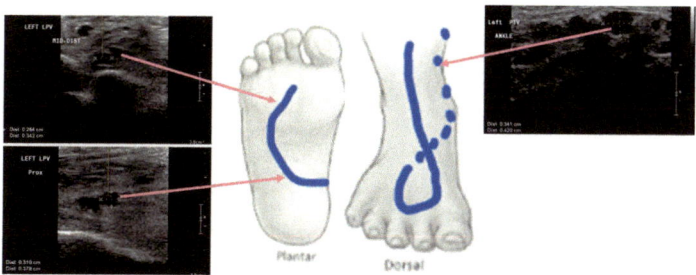

Fig. 8.2 Preoperative measurements and characteristics of LPV and PTV

foot while characterizing tortuosity, pathology, and/or prominent valves of the LPV (Fig. 8.2)
- Mark potential LPV access points as distal as possible of the dominant lateral plantar vein
• Note if the PTV, GSV, or any of the pedal veins are thrombosed or absent

8.3   Recommended Products

• Sterile pneumatic tourniquet
   - Inflated to 100–120 mmHg
   - Alternative: Sterile Esmarch close to the ankle
• 4F Pedal MicroAccess kit with echogenic needle
• Soft tip wires:
   - 0.018 × 180/300 cm; nitinol or steel with shapeable tip
   - Angled or J-tip to avoid tributary veins
• Vasodilators
   - Nitroglycerine, papaverine, or verapamil
• 4F sheath for venous catheter (V-Ceiver)

Procedural Steps

9

Anahita Dua, Sara Rose-Sauld,
and Lindsey Ferraro

Adequate day of case preparation for the TADV procedure is a crucial element for success throughout each procedural step. The initial step involves gaining pedal venous access in the LPV under ultrasound guidance. Although more difficult, use of the tibial vein at the ankle is a viable secondary access point if pedal access cannot be obtained. Following successful venous access, femoral access is obtained at the common femoral. With both access points achieved, the arteriovenous crossing process can commence. The arterial catheter crossing needle is advanced into the venous catheter mesh snare once alignment is achieved. Prior to stenting, all valves must be effaced. The stenting process begins at the ankle with extension stents and ends with the crossing stent. Post-stent angiography is suggested to confirm a pedal loop. Throughout this chapter, helpful "watchouts" and tips are given for each step of the procedure.

A. Dua (✉)
Vascular Surgery, Massachusetts General Hospital/Harvard Medical
School, Boston, MA, USA
e-mail: adua1@mgh.harvard.edu

S. Rose-Sauld
Podiatry, Massachusetts General Hospital, Boston, MA, USA
e-mail: SROSE-SAULD@mgh.harvard.edu

L. Ferraro
Vascular Surgery, Massachusetts General Hospital, Boston, MA, USA
e-mail: LTFERRARO@mgh.harvard.edu

9.1 Case Preparation

- General anesthesia is strongly recommended or conscious sedation with a popliteal block
- Prepare the index limb for standard ipsilateral superficial femoral artery and pedal plantar vein access
- Antibiotics per institutional standard of care
- Standard anticoagulation protocol throughout the procedure with ACT level > 250 s
- Non-sterile ultrasound check for marking of the venous access point
- Circumferentially prep the entire leg
- Drape the leg free and allow room for the tourniquet (Fig. 9.1)
- Place pneumatic tourniquet or sterile Esmarch (Fig. 9.1)
- Leave space for pedal puncture and ultrasound imaging of the foot

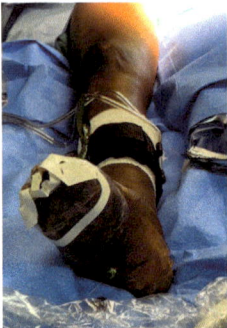 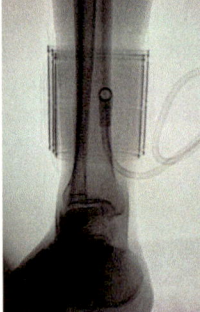 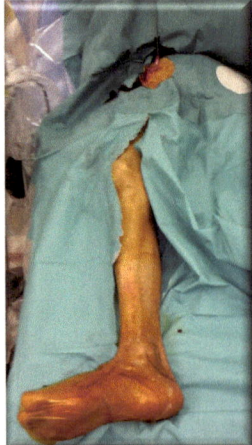

Fig. 9.1 Case preparation

9.2   Pedal Access and Interventional Techniques (Fig. 9.2)

- Recommended equipment:
  - Sterile pneumatic tourniquet
    Can be above the ankle to the mid-calf
    Inflated to 100–120 mmHg
    Alternative: Sterile Esmarch close to the ankle
  - 4F Pedal MicroAccess kit with echogenic needle
  - Soft tip wires:
    0.018 x 180/300 cm; nitinol or steel with shapeable tip
    Angled or J-tip to avoid tributary veins
  - Vasodilators
    Nitroglycerine, papaverine, or verapamil
  - 4F sheath for venous catheter (V-Ceiver)
  - The table in reverse Trendelenburg
- Considerations (Fig. 9.3a, b):
  - Veins are highly compressible
  - Pressure applied with a transducer can easily collapse the vein (Fig. 9.3a)

These valves will be disrupted in the vein chosen to arterialize to direct blood flow to the distal foot.

- Confirmatory venogram (Fig. 9.4)
  - Cuff inflated to 180 or tight sterile Esmarch.
  - Venogram with 0.018 x 300 cm wire in PTV.
  - 20–40 cc heparinized saline injected while the tourniquet is up followed by standard injection of dilute contrast.
- Secondary (Diagnostic) Access: dorsal venogram of medial marginal vein

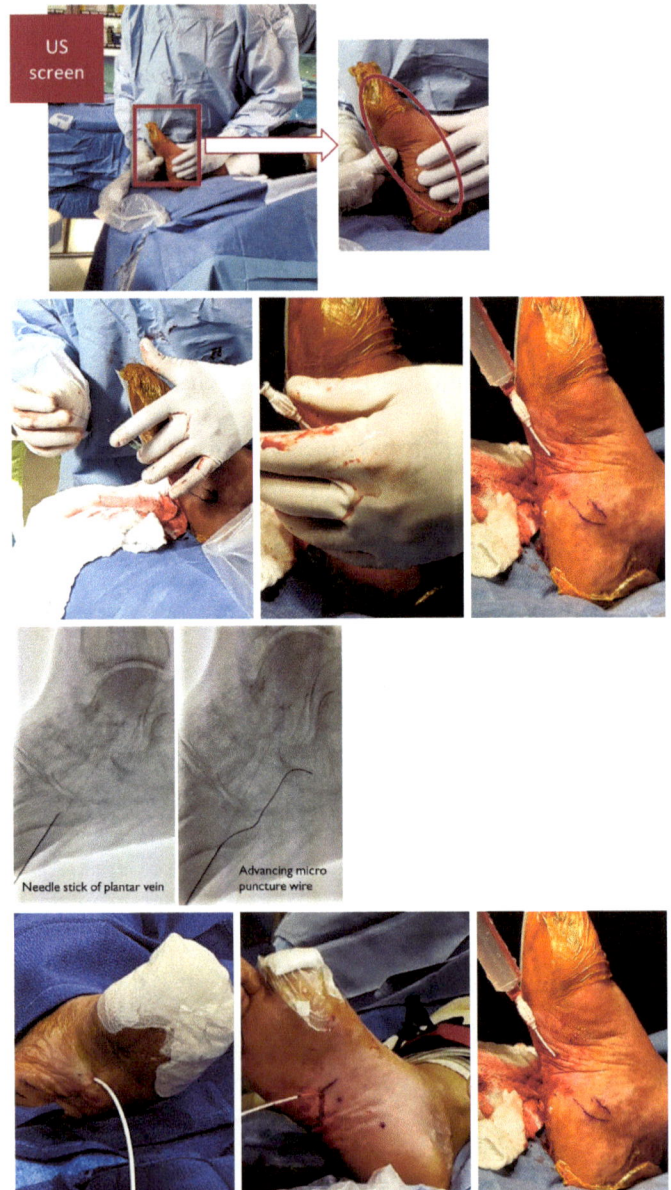

Fig. 9.2 Needle stick of the plantar vein and subsequent micropuncture wire advancement

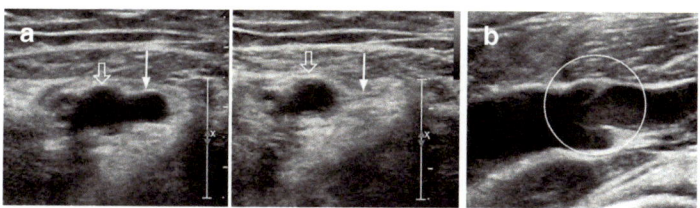

Fig. 9.3 (**a**) In contrast to arteries (open arrows), veins (arrows) have a weaker muscular layer with less elastic walls, and therefore completely collapse when compressed by the transducer. (**b**) Veins contain valves that play an important role in preventing venous reflux

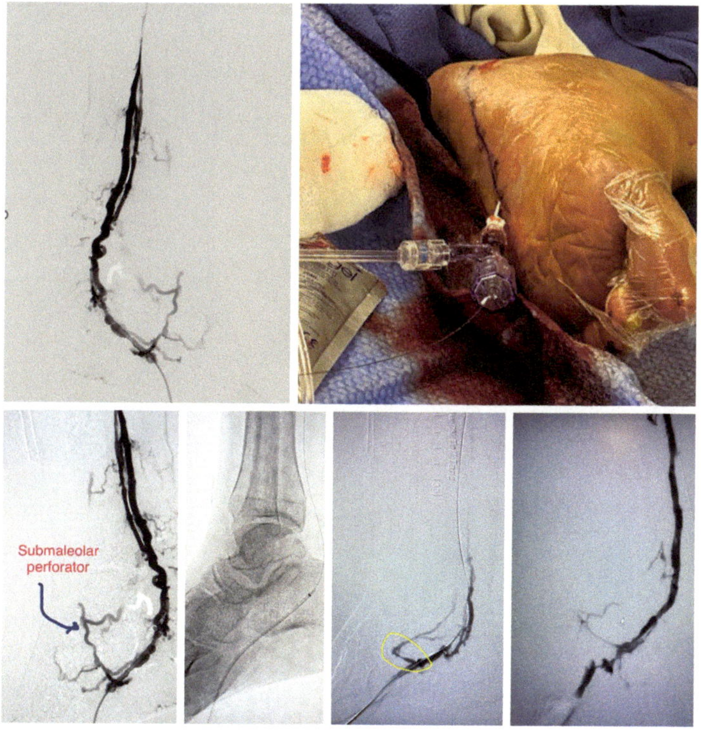

Submaleolar
perforator

Fig. 9.4 Confirmatory venogram is performed after venous access is obtained

- Variant/ tortuous anatomy or 2 unsuccessful LPV access attempts may require additional access to the medial marginal vein for visualization.
- Use the tourniquet at the ankle to increase the pressure in the foot venous system
- Obtain access into the superficial MMV using the micropuncture device (Fig. 9.5)
- Navigate the tip of the introducer toward first toe perforating vein
- A 10–20 cc bolus of heparinized saline followed by a dilute contrast (20 cc bolus at quarter strength) allows for filling of the venous system and visualization without dramatically increasing contrast dosage
- Continue injection until the LPV is visualized (Fig. 9.5)

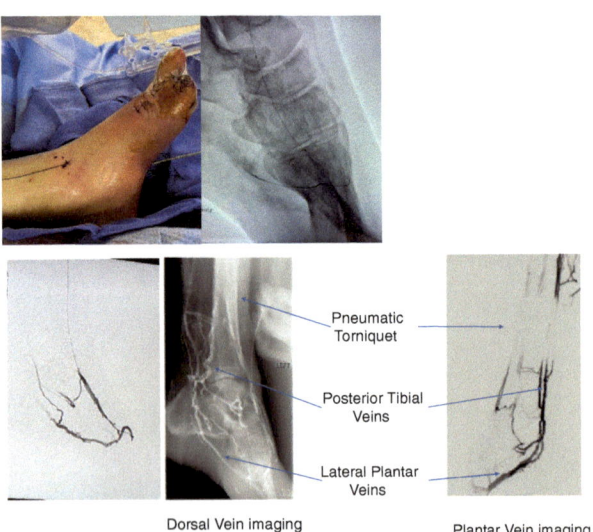

Dorsal Vein imaging   Plantar Vein imaging

Fig. 9.5 Visualization of the lateral plantar veins

9.3   Venous Access Watch Outs and Tips

- Watch outs
    - LPV runs 1.5–3 cm deep. Do not confuse it with the medial plantar vein that runs medial to the midline of the foot
    - Veins exist in paired systems: One vein may be larger than the other and more desirable for intervention (Fig. 9.6)
    - Valves

        Retrograde venous wire cannulation can be difficult due to valves. This can cause damage or perforation to the vein, and retrograde cannulation should be minimized.

        Traversing valves against the flow can be traumatic and can result in diversion into tributaries. This access is typically performed when accessing the medial marginal vein. Traversing valves with the flow is ideal but care should still be taken when navigating the wire through valves. This is the reason lateral plantar vein access is preferred.

        If access is made into a valve, retrieve the needle and pick another access point
    - Thinner media layer

        Veins are thinner and more fragile than arteries and can be easily damaged during wire and device manipulation.
    - Vessel perforation

        A common complication when performing retrograde (against the flow) vein access

        A soft center-seeking wire is preferred with antegrade access, and a stiffer angled wire is preferred for retrograde access
    - Spasm

        Device manipulation can cause veins to spasm and can negatively impact a procedure and patency

        Vasodilators are useful to relieve venous spasm within the limits of the patient's blood pressure

        Keep foot warm

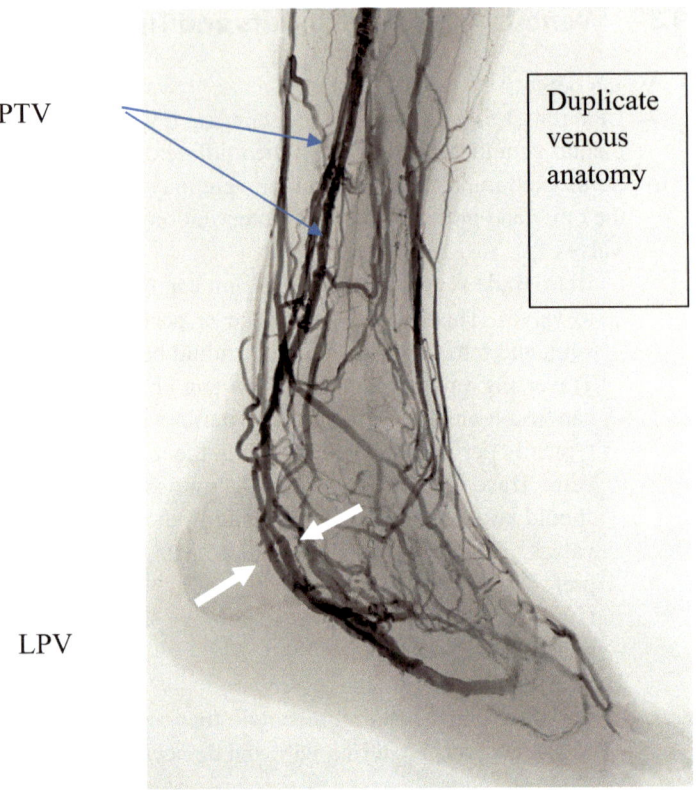

Fig. 9.6 Duplicate venous anatomy

- Multiple crossing points and collaterals may lead to unintentional wire crossing of venous branches (Fig. 9.7)

    During the procedure, the operator confirms the venous wire is in a parallel branch of the PTV at the desired AV crossing.

    Two indications:

    The wire was difficult to advance beyond the popliteal
    In relation to the PTA wire, it appears to "spiral" around the PTA

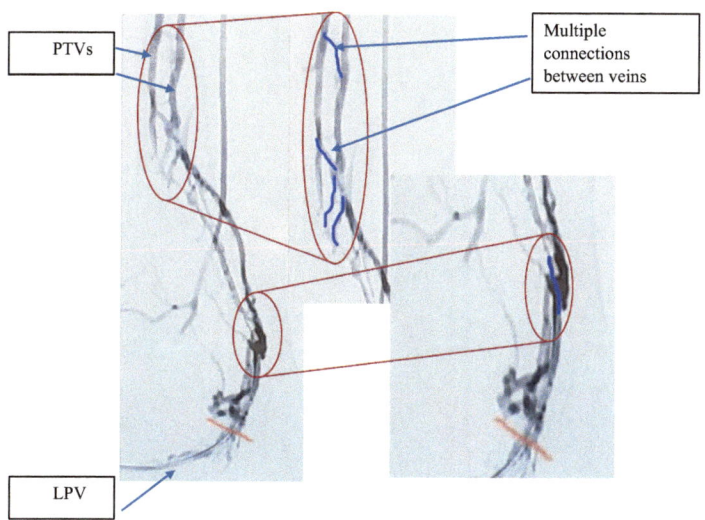

Fig. 9.7 Multiple connections between veins

> Non-linear direction of the venous wire could indicate bridge crossing
>
> By pulling back the wire, the desired PTV is correctly wired (Fig. 9.8)

- Secondary access: target tibial venous access (Fig. 9.9)
  - If unable to gain successful pedal access revert to tibial venous access at the ankle
  - Duplex ultrasound-guided puncture (recommend 1″ above ankle)
  - Introducer and 0.018″ wire advanced to above planned crossing point
  - Consider pre-dilation with 3–4 mm PTA if hard to advance
  - Insert 4F long sheath and dilator
  - NOTE: navigation around the pedal venous loop is considerably more difficult due to valve direction when using this access point.
- Tips and tricks

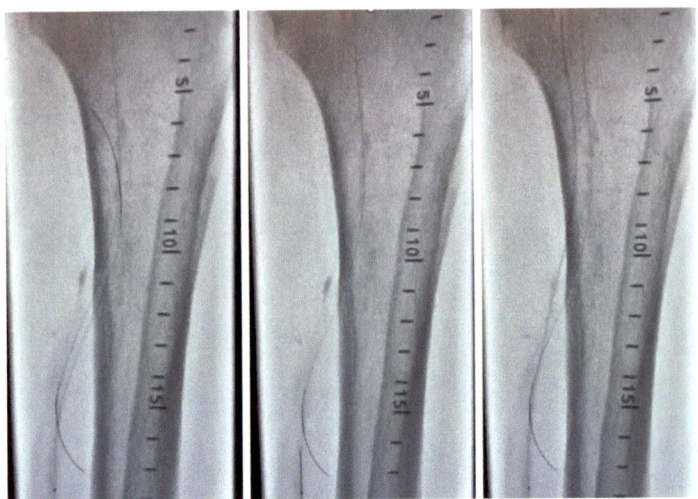

Fig. 9.8 Desired PTV correctly wired after pulling back the wire

- Access as distal as possible
- Recommend a venogram roadmap before wiring to assess the viability of the access point
- Using a shaped wire (j-tip or curved/angled wire tip)
- Administer vasodilators as needed
- Avoid retrograde venous navigation to the degree possible (valves, spasm, perforation, side branches)
- A lateral plantar puncture algorithm (Fig. 9.10) can help guide access points and reduce trauma to the pedal venous system:

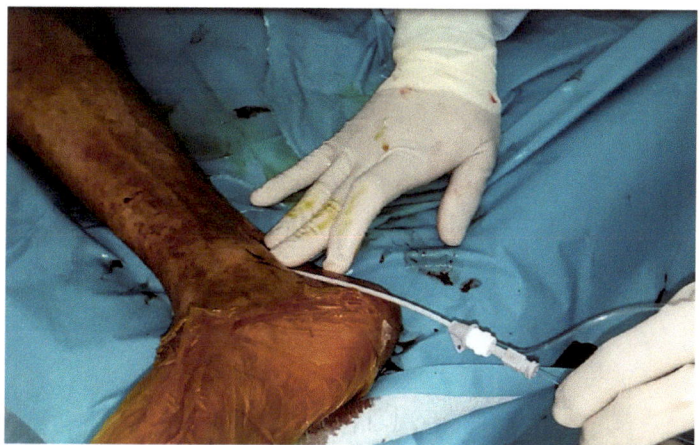

Fig. 9.9 Tibial venous access if unable to achieve pedal venous access

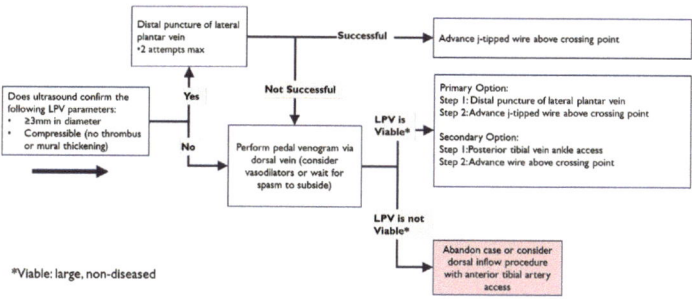

Fig. 9.10 Lateral plantar puncture algorithm

9.4 Femoral Access

- Antegrade approach for access to common femoral (Fig. 9.11)
- Fix all inflow disease in the SFA / POP prior to the TADV procedure
- If stenting is required, recommend stenting post-TADV

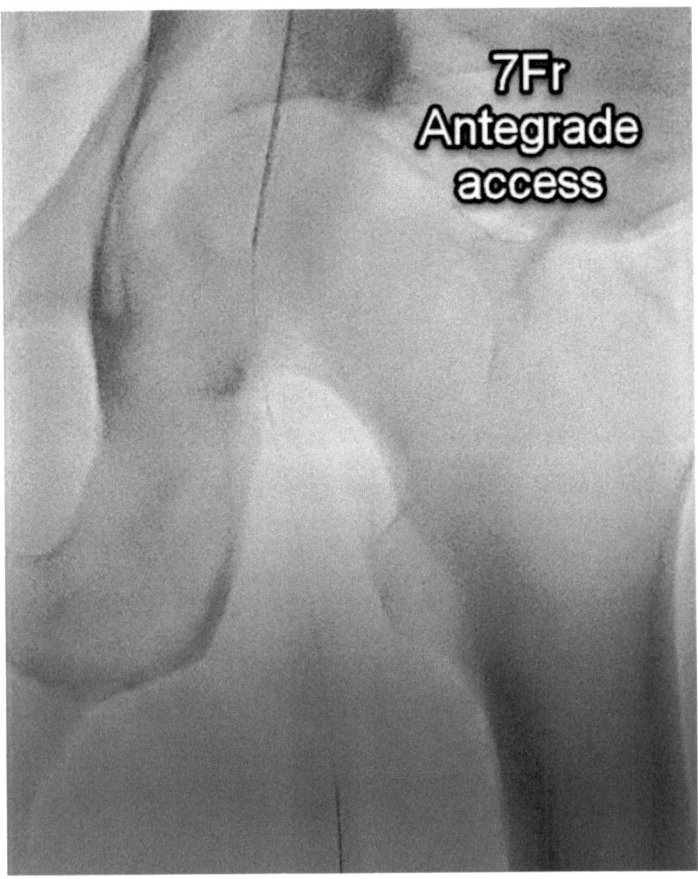

Fig. 9.11 Common femoral access

9.5   Crossing Preparation

- Once access is achieved, visualization and identification of the crossing location can be performed.
  - An 0.014″ guidewire should be placed via the 4F sheath and advanced through the donor vein beyond the desired crossing location

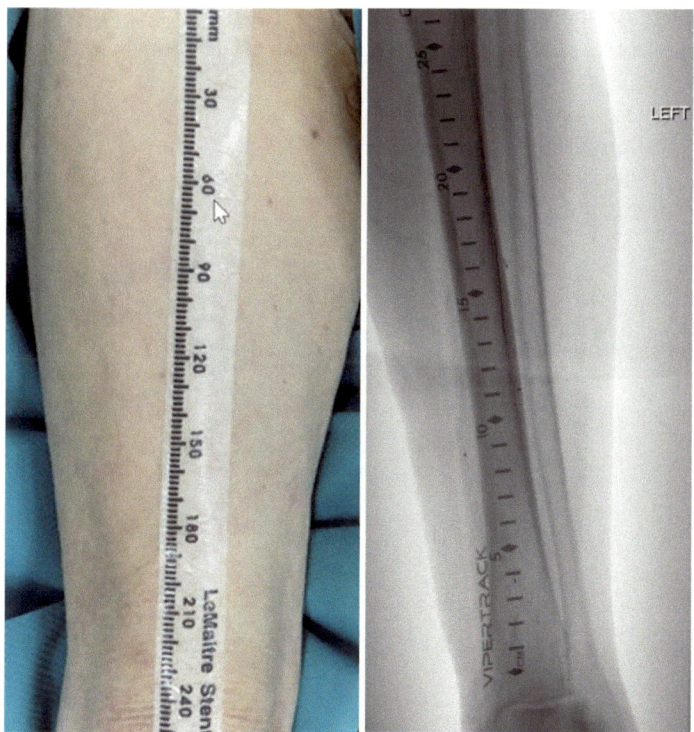

Fig. 9.12 Sterile angiographic ruler

- An 0.014″ guidewire should be placed via the 7F introducer sheath and advanced beyond the target crossing location
- Rotate the angiography unit, so the distance between the two wires at the desired crossing location is maximized
- Apply a sterile angiographic ruler along the lower limb and make sure it does not obscure the sight of the wire. If you use a non-sterile ruler, then place it under the table pad (not ideal) (Fig. 9.12).

- A double injection is recommended to simultaneously image the arterial and venous anatomy to confirm the crossing point (Fig. 9.13).
- The suggested crossing point is a minimum of 2 cm below the ostium of the target artery (PTA, ATA, or Peroneal).
- If possible, avoid covering collaterals to retain distal tibial flow.

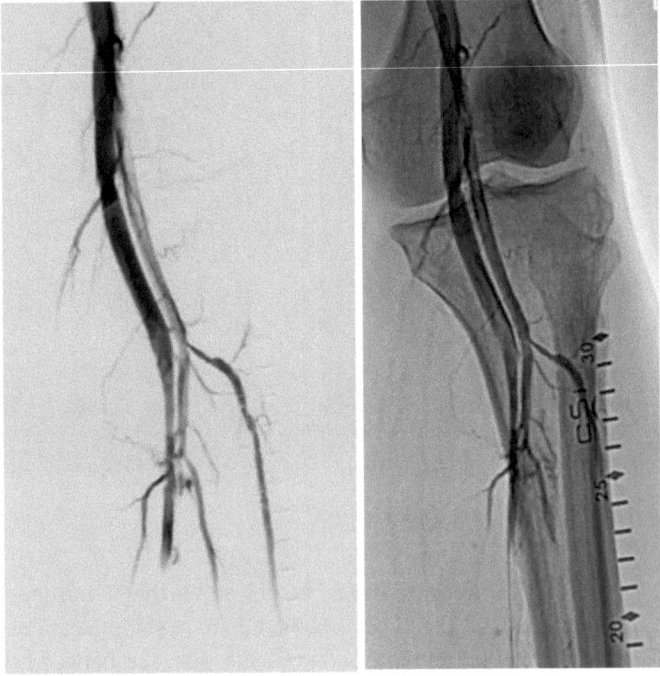

Fig. 9.13 Simultaneous imaging of arterial & venous anatomy

- **NOTE: It is paramount that all native arterial flow to the lower leg be preserved; failure to do so can result in acute ischemia and severe pain native arterial flow will continue to promote viability of the limb post venous arterialization creation and maturation**
- Arteriovenous crossing
  Using LimFlow V'Ceiver:
  - Ensure the venous catheter is flushed and the Tuohy-Borst valve is locked
  - Introduce the catheter over the 0.014″ wire to the desired crossing location (repeat double-injection angiography as needed)
  - Deploy the mesh snare:
      Unlock Tuohy-Borst valve
      Pin the inner core shaft/guidewire luer with the right hand and keep fixed
      Pull the Tuohy-Borst valve with the left hand toward the right
  - Lock Tuohy-Borst valve
  - Do not reposition the V-Ceiver with the mesh deployed; recapture the snare before adjusting the catheter position
  - Using LimFlow ARC:
  - Ensure the device is flushed, and the crossing needle is completely inside the catheter
  - Introduce the arterial catheter over the 0.014″ guidewire using the monorail lumen
  - Advance the catheter until the needle port is at the intended crossing point (repeat double-injection angiography as needed) and parallel to the venous catheter
  - The needle exit port is proximal to the guiding marker ~22 mm from the tip

Figure 9.14 load a recommended 0.014″ 300 cm (Thruway Boston Scientific, Nitrex—Medtronic, Runthrough—Terumo) crossing wire into the guidewire lumen.

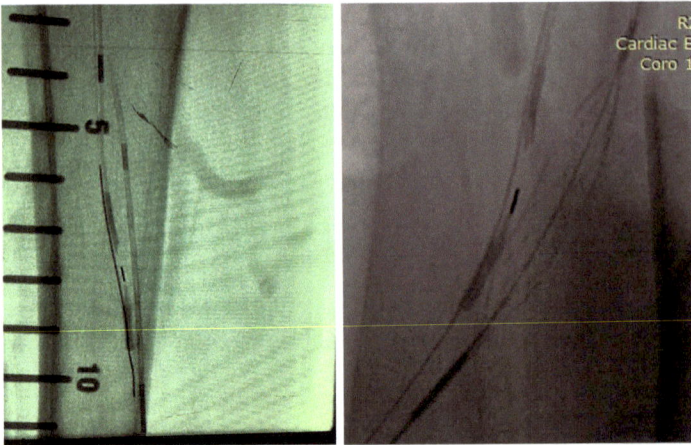

Fig. 9.14 Crossing wire in lumen of guidewire

9.6 Artery to Vein Alignment: C-Arm Positioning

Primary Alignment Method: Eclipse View and 90° Offset

- Rotate C-arm until the arterial catheter wire near the marker band and the venous catheter wire at the midpoint of the deployed mesh are directly overlapping (eclipsed)
- Rotate the C-arm 90°
- You are now viewing the crossing plane

Secondary Alignment Method: Maximum Distance

- Rotate C-arm until the arterial catheter wire near the marker band and the venous catheter wire at the midpoint of the deployed snare are at the greatest distance from each other
- You are now viewing the crossing plane (Fig. 9.15)
- **Tip:** Once optimal alignment is achieved, do not move catheters proximally or distally before crossing

After Confirming the Correct C-Arm Position

- Align the arterial catheter (ARC) and venous catheter (V-Ceiver) longitudinally
- Position the arterial catheter radiopaque marker so that it is aligned longitudinally with the center of the mesh (Fig. 9.15)
- Using the radiopaque marker, rotate the arterial catheter to align it to the venous catheter.

Crossing Needle Deployment: With the Arterial Catheter (ARC) Aligned to the Target Vein

- Retract the 0.014" OTW from the snare mesh to provide more space to capture the crossing wire
- Ensure the arterial catheter is loaded with a recommended crossing 0.014" guidewire
- Advance the arterial catheter(ARC) crossing needle directly into the mesh
- Tip: Small movements of the venous catheter mesh can help to confirm needle and/or wire entry into the vein. Distal/proximal motion or rotation has worked

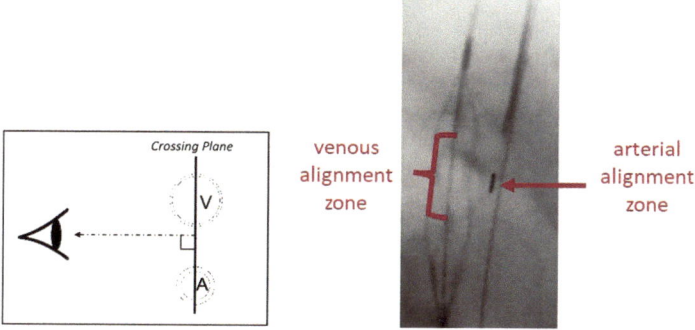

Fig. 9.15   Crossing plane and venous and arterial alignment zone

Artery to Vein Crossing: Advance Crossing Guidewire (Fig. 9.16)

- Advance the floppy portion of the crossing guidewire through the needle into the mesh
  - Snaring the stiff portion of the crossing wire may cause excessive damage to the catheter
- Do not retract the crossing wire with the needle deployed
  - Retract the needle first, THEN retract the crossing wire
- Prior to snaring, retract the crossing needle fully into the Arterial Catheter (ARC)
- **Tip**: Only target the central portion of the wire's radiopaque tip for snaring. This is the most flexible portion of the wire.

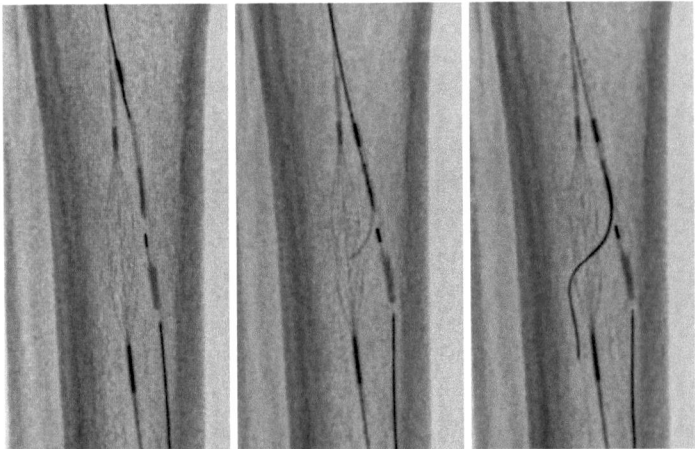

Fig. 9.16 Crossing guidewire advanced through the needle and into the mesh

Artery to Vein Crossing: Guidewire Capture (Fig. 9.17)

- Target the central portion of the radiopaque wire tip
- Snare the wire by pinning the guidewire port and carefully advancing the outer sheath. This re-constrains the snare mesh along with the crossing wire.
- It is normal to feel some resistance. The distal tip of the wire is bent and constrained with the mesh to a small diameter.
- If excessive force is felt, **STOP**. The wire is secured in the catheter, so it is OK to retract the catheter with the mesh slightly exposed (see right image). Better this than break the wire.
- With wire captured, **Tighten the Tuohy-Borst Before Withdrawing**

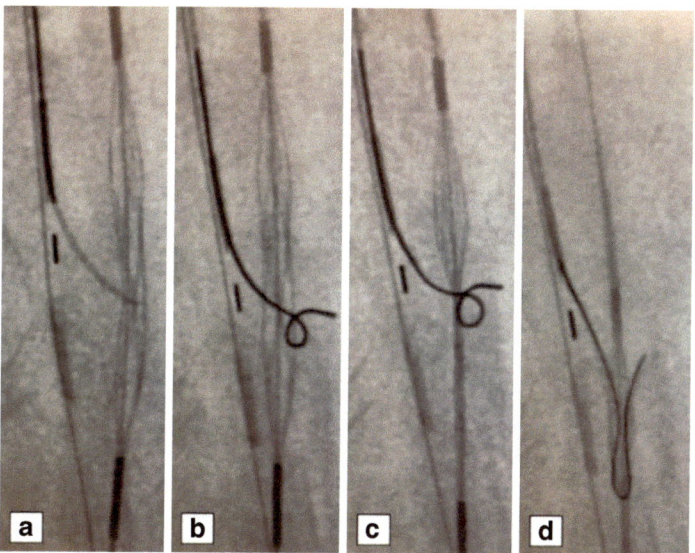

Fig. 9.17 Guidewire capture. (**a**) Crossing needle protruding into snare basket. (**b**) Delivery of the 0.14 wire into the snare basket. (**c**) Capture of the 0.14 wire by the snare. (**d**) Retrieval of the wire to gain through and through access from the pedal access point

- Withdraw the venous catheter with wire out of the venous access point while simultaneously feeding the wire from the arterial access point.
- **Note:** Wire capture is possible without fully retracting the venous catheter (V-Ceiver) mesh

Artery to Vein Crossing: Guidewire Externalization

The venous catheter (V-Ceiver) and crossing wire are withdrawn from the body through the venous access point:

- Ensure you have adequate crossing wire length out of the venous access
- Retract the outer sheath to expose the snare mesh and wire
- It is normal for the wire to be kinked, but not broken
- Secure the newly externalized 0.014″ wire using a hemostat or torque handle to trap the wire outside the pedal access sheath
- With 0.014″ wire access across the AV fistula, carefully withdraw the arterial catheter (ARC) from the arterial access
- Secure the distal (venous access) end of the crossing wire before removing the catheter
  - A hemostat fixed to the wire is recommended

Dilating the Conduit (Fig. 9.18)

- Use a short 3.5mm or 4.0 mm balloon to dilate the arteriovenous crossing point
  - Balloon sizing depends on the arterial diameter of the tapered crossing stent
  - It is important to confirm the crossing location by visualizing the pinched area in the balloon and coregister it with the radiopaque marker in the field of view.

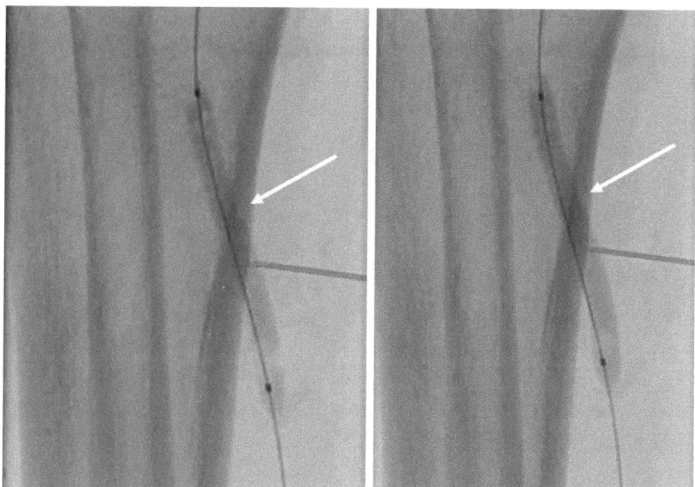

Fig. 9.18 Dilating the conduit

9.7   Crossing Watch Outs and Tips

- Wire snagged into a side branch
- Insufficient wire length for support
- Calcium doesn't allow the support catheter to pass
- Avoid over-manipulation of the retrograde sheath as it will traumatize the vein and make a bigger hole. A small knock at the pedal access site can relieve strain on this access point.
- Use a fresh 0.014 crossing wire
- Use a straight tip on the wire
- Use a hemostat to compress the skin puncture site
- Dorsiflex the ankle to straighten the veins

9.8   Valve Effacement

- Exchange the "Through-and-through" wire to an 0.018″ platform
- Ensure that both lumen (wire and cage) of the valvulotome catheter are flushed.

- Confirm that the cutting cage is in the "closed" configuration before introduction into the sheath introducer
- The Tuohy-Borst valve has to be locked to avoid the cage opening at an unintended location.
- Introduce the valvulotome catheter over the 0.018″ guidewire
- When using LimFlow VECTOR™
  - Exchange the "Through-and-through" wire to an 0.018″ platform
  - Ensure that both lumen (wire and cage) of the valvulotome catheter are flushed.
  - Confirm that the cutting cage is in the "closed"-configuration before introduction into the sheath introducer
  - The Tuohy-Borst valve has to be locked to avoid the cage opening at an unintended location.
  - Introduce the valvulotome catheter over the 0.018″ guidewire
  - Ensure all valves are effaced before deploying stents (Fig. 9.19)
  - Additional tools to efface valves
      High-pressure balloons
      Cutting/Scoring balloons
  - Do not inflate balloons over nominal pressure in areas not covered by a stent graft
  - Aggressive angioplasty distal to the stent may result in early occlusion
  - NOTE: in the calf and around the ankle have to be resolved with more aggressive technologies before stenting, e.g. cutting balloon or high-pressure balloon

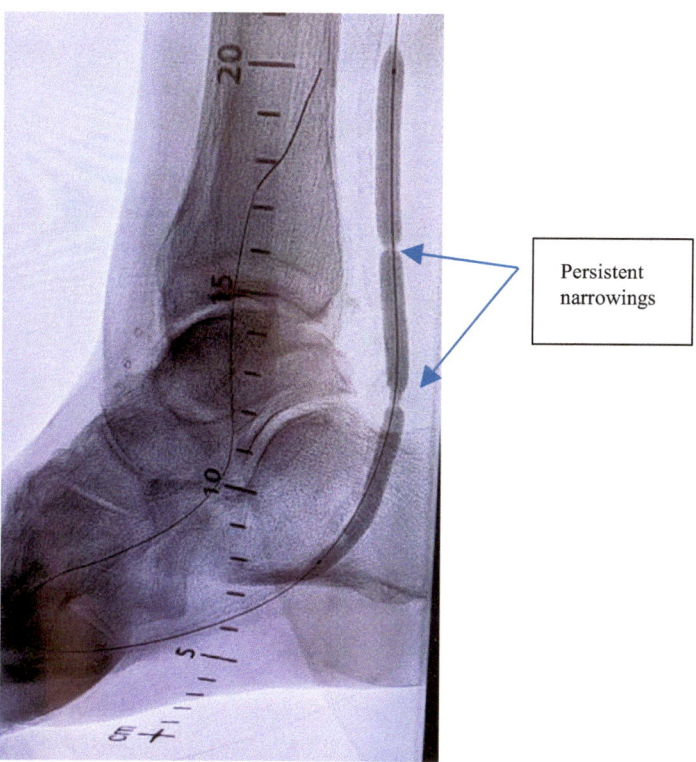

Fig. 9.19 Persistent narrowing (venous valves)

9.9   Stent Deployment (Fig. 9.20)

- Estimate stent length based on angiographic tape length and decide which configuration of stents to use
- Begin by deploying extension stents starting at the ankle
- Deploy crossing stent last
  - NOTE: LimFlow system includes a tapered crossing stent to allow appropriate adaptation to the vessel size difference in the arterial and venous crossover, good apposition, and appropriate flow pattern. **The use of a non-tapered stent may introduce complications in the arteriovenous crossing**

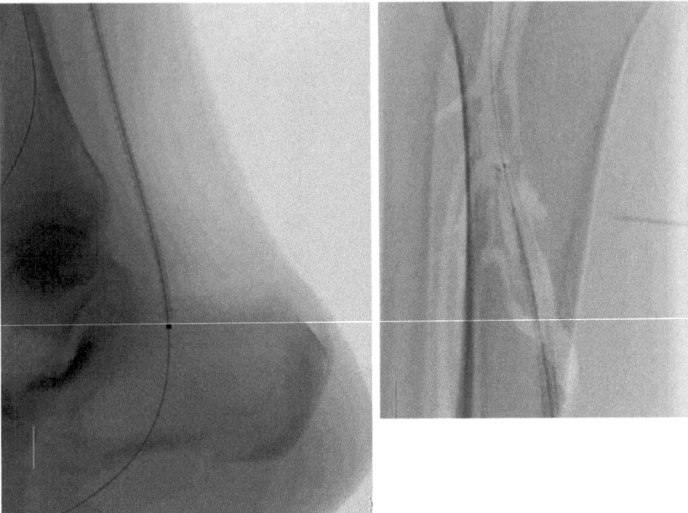

Fig. 9.20 Stent deployment

- Land most distal extension stent at or above the calcaneus
- Require approximately 1 cm of overlap between stents (3–4 Stent Struts)
- Land tapered crossing stent approximately 2 cm into the artery (6–8 stent struts)
- Post dilatation, recommend a 5 mm balloon inflated to nominal
- In the proximal end of the crossing stent, use a balloon sized to the tibial artery
- Aggressive angioplasty distal to the stent may result in early occlusion

Pedal Loop Wiring

- Post-stent angiography may confirm pedal loop
- If a complete outflow loop is unsatisfactory:
- Introduce a second 0.014″ or 0.018″ wire from the 7Fr arterial access

- Advance wire through the new TADV stent into the LPV beyond the pedal sheath access
- Remove the externalized wire from the pedal sheath
- Using a micro-support catheter, advance the new wire around the LPV, into the metatarsal perforator, and the GSV, SSV, or ATV
- Consider using a 3 mm or 4 mm balloon with very low pressure to support hemostasis at the venous access after removing the venous sheath.
- The valves of the LPV should be disrupted. Reintroduction of the antegrade over-the-wire valvulotome can be done through the arterial access. Unsheath the valvulotome distal to the TADV stent and advance the device until the tip starts to deflect in the metatarsal perforator (Fig. 9.21).

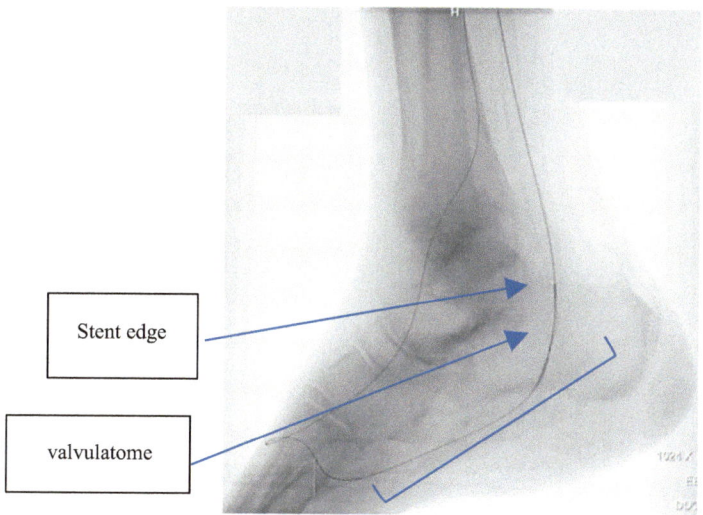

Fig. 9.21 LPV valve disruption

End of Case

- Look for complete arch formation
- Must have outflow
- Recommend taking multiple views (AP and lateral) and ensuring angiograms are recorded to allow for comparison during follow-up. The final angiograms should be done with the wire out to ensure all valves have been rendered incompetent.
- Criteria for acute success include an appropriate seal and connection that has been created between the donor artery and the donor vein with arterial flow moving distally through the end of the stent into the mid to distal foot and, ideally, the metatarsal area. The venous outflow should be continuous with very little to no stagnant flow in its path. The remaining native tibial arteries should flow with little diminished flow (Fig. 9.22).

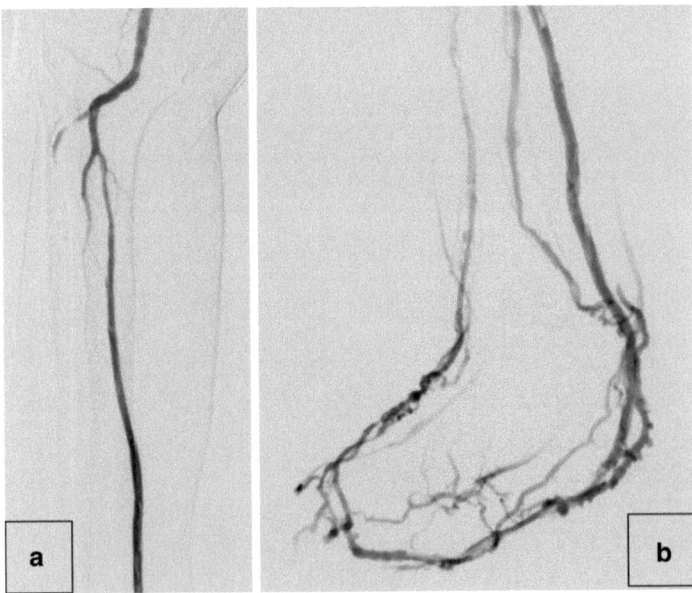

Fig. 9.22 (**a**) Demonstrates successful posterior tibial artery to posterior tibial vein TADV creation and arteriovenous seal by the tapered stent graft. (**b**) Demonstrates flow to the metatarsal perforator and appropriate outflow through the dorsal venous system

Immediate Postoperative Care

10

Anahita Dua, Sara Rose-Sauld, and Lindsey Ferraro

Immediately following the TADV procedure, patients can experience pain and edema, which should be closely monitored to identify any signs of more significant pain or wound deterioration that could be indicative of an underlying cause. This time point is essential to ensure patency and avoid thrombosis. Therefore, a post-operative Doppler ultrasound should be performed to confirm adequate blood flow, and an additional vascular DUS should be conducted post-op to obtain baseline volume flow rates. For patients with stable wounds, wound care post-TADV should remain the same and continued close surveillance is essential to reduce the occurrence of necrosis.

A. Dua (✉) · L. Ferraro
Division of Vascular and Endovascular Surgery, Massachusetts General Hospital/Harvard Medical School, Boston, MA, USA
e-mail: ADUA1@mgh.harvard.edu; LTFERRARO@mgh.harvard.edu

S. Rose-Sauld
Podiatry, Massachusetts General Hospital, Boston, MA, USA
e-mail: SROSE-SAULD@mgh.harvard.edu

10.1   Expectations After TADV

- Edema can occur in the treated limb after TADV and typically resolves within 3–4 weeks
- Acceleration in healing typically occurs 4–6 weeks after the procedure and is likely due to maturation of the arterialization, wound conditions may deteriorate during this time. It is important to note that healing may take longer than 4–6 weeks if there are surgical interventions including debridement or minor amputation during this timfce.
- Any significant changes/deterioration of the wound, include increasing pain and skin discoloration, warrant second look consideration of non-nutritive flow or arterial steal.

10.2   Post-Procedure Care

- Anti-coagulation and anti-platelet per institution standard of care
- Pain management per institution standard of care
  - **Potential sources**
       Periprocedural—soon after TADV, 24–48 h post procedure
       Ischemia
  - **Pain management options**
       Regional anesthetic
       Oral/IV systemic medication
  - **Severe pain or pain that has not resolved within 24–48 h should raise concern for new ischemia (arterial steal) and should be investigated**
- Edema may occur postoperatively, treat per the institution's standard of care
  - Recommend elevating leg after procedure
  - May use compression to treat edema
       Light compression, not higher than 20 mmHg with either anti-thrombotic stockings Class I or bandages with a defined pressure application, e.g., Profore light, Coban light

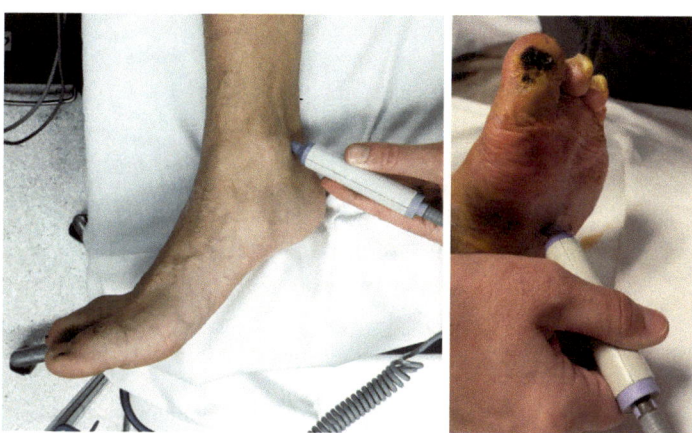

Fig. 10.1 Continuous wave Doppler

- Continuous **wave Doppler (bedside pencil Doppler)**
  - Listen at ankle level where the stent graft terminates (Fig. 10.1)
  - Characterize sound by pitch and cycle (high vs. low resistance)
  - Listen to flow along LPV plantar course
  - Listen to medial marginal and DP vein outflow on the dorsal foot
        Looking for acute thrombosis and to verify patency
- Vascular DUS from groin to foot
  - Volume flow rates based on duplex
  - Recommend 100–300 ml/min
  - Focus on mid-stent, stent outflow, and in the lateral plantar vein
  - Note: May be difficult to visualize through covered stents immediately after implantation, if that is the case, then visualize proximal and distal to stents to confirm patency and attempt a duplex of the stent in the coming days
  - **Consider arteriogram if there is a loss of flow or dramatic negative change in flow**
- Routine surveillance of the wound and index limb

10.3   Wound Care

- Essentially wound care does not change after TADV as long as the wound stays stable. However, keep in mind that patients will often convert from wet to dry gangrene so frequent surveillance is essential to minimizing tissue necrosis due to infection
- The biggest difference is that open transmetatarsal (TMA) amputations are performed instead of closing the TMA with a flap at the original operation
- Betadine-soaked gauze and dry dressing if stable, dry gangrene
- Resection of infected tissue if infected
  - Offload heels while in bed even if no heel ulcers are present.

Anticoagulation

Post procedure the patient is maintained on dual antiplatelet therapy typically aspirin and clopidogrel.

Post-TADV Care Plan

11

Anahita Dua, Sara Rose-Sauld, and Lindsey Ferraro

The first 3 months following the TADV procedure hold immense importance in determining long-term success of the procedure. To ensure optimal outcomes, patients should be enrolled in a wound care clinic and undergo regular duplex ultrasound evaluations. By conducting vigilant wound surveillance, the care team has the opportunity for early assessment and treatment of any potential issues. This early-intensive approach followed by our clinic allows arterialization adequate time to flourish with minimal interferences.

The TADV procedure is the starting point for a patient's journey to complete wound healing. The days, weeks, and months after the procedure are key to the success story. Patient care within the first 6 weeks is the most important and resource intensive, from both an intellectual and procedural aspect. In the following chapters, we will dive into the various aspects of creating a successful post-TADV care plan, including circuit and wound surveillance and treatment options for issues that may arise.

A. Dua (✉) · L. Ferraro
Division of Vascular and Endovascular Surgery, Massachusetts General Hospital/Harvard Medical School, Boston, MA, USA
e-mail: ADUA1@mgh.harvard.edu; LTFERRARO@mgh.harvard.edu

S. Rose-Sauld
Podiatry, Massachusetts General Hospital, Boston, MA, USA
e-mail: SROSE-SAULD@mgh.harvard.edu

© The Author(s), under exclusive license to Springer Nature Switzerland AG 2023
A. Dua et al. (eds.), *The Massachusetts General Hospital Approach to Transcatheter Arterialization of the Deep Veins for Advanced Limb Salvage*, https://doi.org/10.1007/978-3-031-37510-1_11

Within our institution, we focus our intensity of effort within the first 3 months, with weekly wound clinic visits and frequent (approximately monthly) DUS of the circuit. This allows us to properly stage any extensive podiatric or wound work that needs to occur and perform circuit maturation procedures as appropriate to ensure continued adequate blood flow for remodeling to occur.

For those patients without active wounds, it is still important to be vigilant with circuit observation and preventative checks of the foot to confirm the tissue's health.

Acutely, post-procedure care planning includes:

- Manage underlying pathology
- Plan maintenance care
- Implement local wound care
- Modify the care pathway and refer if necessary to specialists
- Educate patient/family on the standard of care, including the potential for the need for maintenance procedures
- Discharge or transition to maintenance treatment to prevent recurrent issues

In the long term, the care algorithm that we implement is as follows in Fig. 11.1

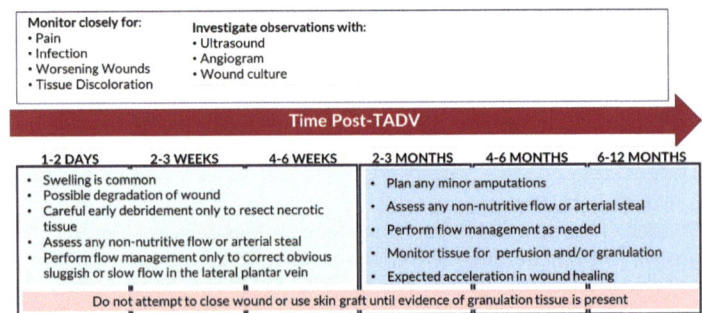

Fig. 11.1 Care algorithm post-TADV

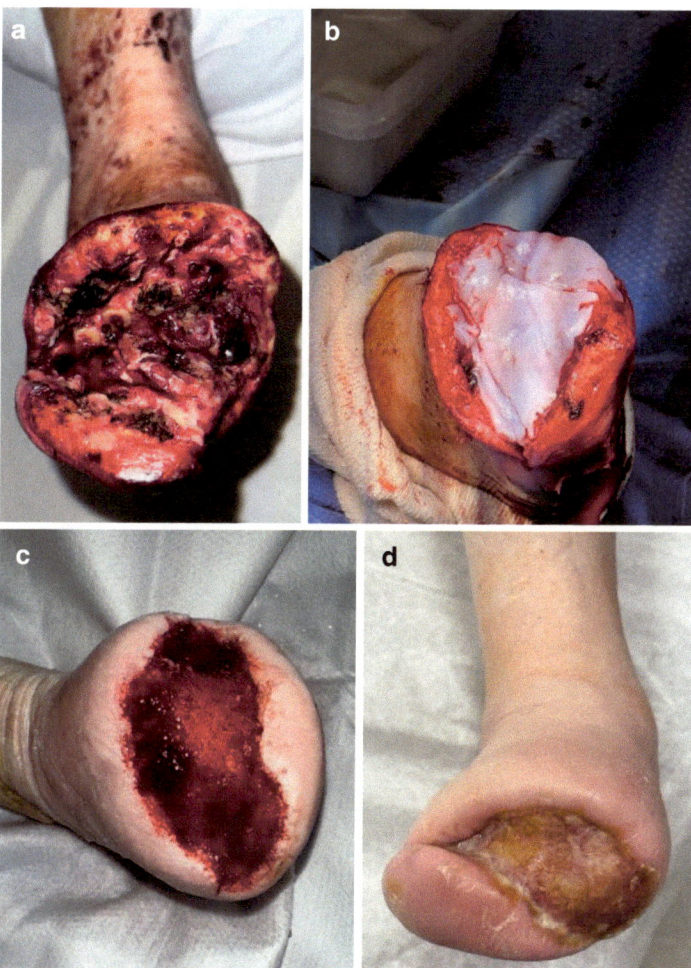

Fig. 11.2 (**a**) Open TMA being careful not to injure the pedal venous loop. (**b**) Open TMA may be covered with skin substitutes with VAC placement 5 days post initial procedure if not ready for a split thickness skin graft. (**c**) Once the wound bed demonstrated granulation, a split thickness skin graft may be placed for coverage. (**d**) Split thickness skin graft placement over TMA site

- At the 3-month mark the patient may be considered for an open TMA if the DVA circuit has been adequately maintained in this time.
- A guillotine TMA is performed taking special care not to injure the venous pedal loop circuit (Fig. 11.2a).
- We prefer not to place a VAC on the open area at the initial surgical procedure as this may result in skin necrosis.
- On post-operative day 5, a VAC may be placed at 75 mmHg of suction over a skin substitute though this is not a requirement—if there is concern for residual infection antibiotics are continued in this time (Fig. 11.2b).
- Once the wound has demonstrated the ability to develop healthy granulation tissue, a split thickness skin graft may be placed (Fig. 11.2c, d).

Part IV

Post-procedure Care and Maintenance

Imaging the TADV Circuit

12

Lindsey Ferraro, Sara Rose-Sauld,
and Anahita Dua

Discussed in prior chapters, a pre-discharge post-operative duplex ultrasound provides baseline values for comparison at subsequent stages post-TADV. The duplex exams should be completed at 2–4-week intervals for the first two months post-operatively to ensure patency. By obtaining volume flow rate, stenosis, and toe/brachial index measurements, clinicians can evaluate graft patency. Arterial duplex and toe/brachial index interpretation for TADV requires knowledge of measurement ranges and proper technique, which are outlined below.

12.1 Duplex Ultrasound Surveillance

(a) Duplex exams are performed at regular intervals to assess graft patency and identify potential issues.
(b) Obtain the first duplex before discharge, if possible
(c) Serial duplex every 2–4 weeks for the first 8 weeks

L. Ferraro · A. Dua (✉)
Division of Vascular and Endovascular Surgery, Massachusetts General Hospital/Harvard Medical School, Boston, MA, USA
e-mail: LTFERRARO@mgh.harvard.edu; ADUA1@mgh.harvard.edu

S. Rose-Sauld
Podiatry, Massachusetts General Hospital, Boston, MA, USA
e-mail: SROSE-SAULD@mgh.harvard.edu

(d) Establish baseline Volume Flow (VF) rates post-TADV
  - Common femoral artery (CFA) through popliteal level obtain a standard arterial duplex with PSV/EDV
  - Obtain VF rates through the inflow, stent and into outflow arterialized vein.
  - The ideal VF rate through stents and arterialized vein is 100–300 ml/min (for the first 6 month)
  - Post-op TADV waveform should be hyperemic (multiphasic components all above baseline) starting in femoral vessels
  - Provide a visual assessment of potential residual valves or stealing vessels in the foot that may need treatment

12.2 Limitations

(a) Presence of open wounds, burns, casts, or surgical dressings
(b) The inability of the patient to cooperate for exam/limited mobility/patient body habitus

12.3 Equipment

(a) Duplex imaging equipment with various transducer capabilities including a linear 7–9 MHz and linear 8–18i MHz (hockey stick probe)

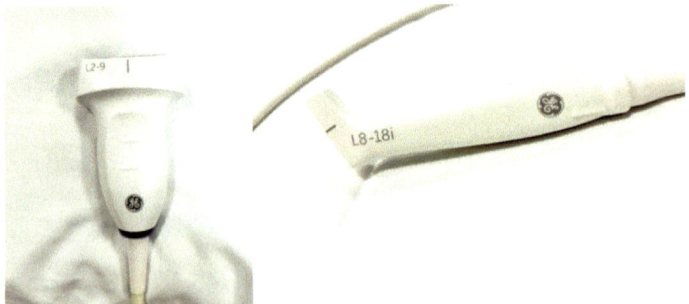

12.4   Patient Prep

(a) Introduction to the patient, verify patient information, and a brief explanation of what the exam will entail
(b) Obtain any pertinent patient history
(c) Have the patient remove any pants, socks, and shoes.
(d) Position the patient in the supine position on the table, drape the patient to maintain privacy, and unwrap any dressings that may be present on the patient
(e) Once the patient's foot is unwrapped, have the patient externally rotate the patient's leg on the exam table that is in a slight reverse Trendelenburg position.

12.5   Procedure

(a) Evaluation of the TADV circuit
   • Equipment gain and display settings should be optimized to provide the best possible grayscale images. Color duplex is utilized to assist in identifying vessels and flow disturbances
   • A lower extremity arterial duplex evaluation must be done to evaluate arterial flow from the groin through the graft to the outflow Lateral Plantar Vein (LPV).
   • The arteries are evaluated in a long axis with grayscale and/or color duplex and spectral pulse wave Doppler
   • Pulse wave Doppler must be obtained in the sagittal plane at an angle of ≤ 60 degrees, keeping the cursor aligned parallel with the flow.
   • Inflow and outflow are assessed with color duplex and pulsed wave Doppler.
   • Flow volumes are also assessed from the inflow, through the graft, and all outflow vessels.
   • A stenotic lesions can be identified by color aliasing and increased velocity.
(b) Evaluation of the digits (if applicable)

- A small (2.5-cm) cuff is placed on the great toe of the TADV foot (or alternate toes due to possible amputation) for a pulse volume recording
  - The cuff is inflated to a maxim of 65–70 mmHg, and waveforms are recorded over three cardiac cycles.
- Photoplethysmography electrodes are attached to the evaluated toe of the TADV foot via adhesive tape/sensor adaptors
  - Photoplethysmographic waveforms are recorded at the level of the toe.
- Resting toe/brachial index is obtained of the TADV foot
  - A cuff is inflated to a pressure of 30 mmHg above an arm systolic pressure or the pressure at which the PPV waveform disappears.
  - The cuff is gradually deflated until the first pulse is seen on the waveforms and the pressure is recorded.

12.6 Required Documentation

(a) All images are stored on PACS.
(b) Arterial duplex
  - Sagittal plane grayscale images and/or color Doppler images must be documented and include the following:
    - Common femoral artery
    - Profunda femoris artery
    - Proximal to distal superficial femoral artery
    - Popliteal artery
    - Distal posterior tibial artery
    - Distal peroneal artery
    - Distal anterior tibial artery
    - TADV stent graft
        Inflow
        Crossing segment
        Mid segment
        Distal anastomosis
        Outflow (LPV)

- Sagittal plane images of pulse wave Doppler samples of peak systolic velocities are obtained in the following:
  - Common femoral artery
  - Profunda femoris artery
  - Proximal to distal superficial femoral artery
  - Popliteal artery
  - Distal posterior tibial artery
  - Distal peroneal artery
  - Distal anterior tibial artery
- Spectral Doppler volume flow rates are obtained in the following:
  - TADV stent graft
    - Inflow
    - Crossing segment
    - Mid segment
    - Distal anastomosis
    - Outflow (LPV)

12.7   Volume Flow Rate Considerations (Fig. 12.1)

(a) Measure diameter intima to intima at the point of insonation. Turn the color flow off to better visualize the vessel wall.

(b) Ensure the diameter measurement is perpendicular to the vessel wall

(c) PW Doppler angle should stay at 60 degrees. Use heel-to-toe "rocking" of the probe to achieve parallel insonation versus decreasing the Doppler angle, if needed.

(d) Increase the sample volume to encompass the entire vessel lumen, going outside the vessel wall if needed.

(e) Use the VF rate measurement package on the US machine, reference the user manual if needed

- Make note of any branches that may be seen around the TADV distal anastomosis (where, diameter, velocities, flow volume). Blood flow takes the path of least resistance,

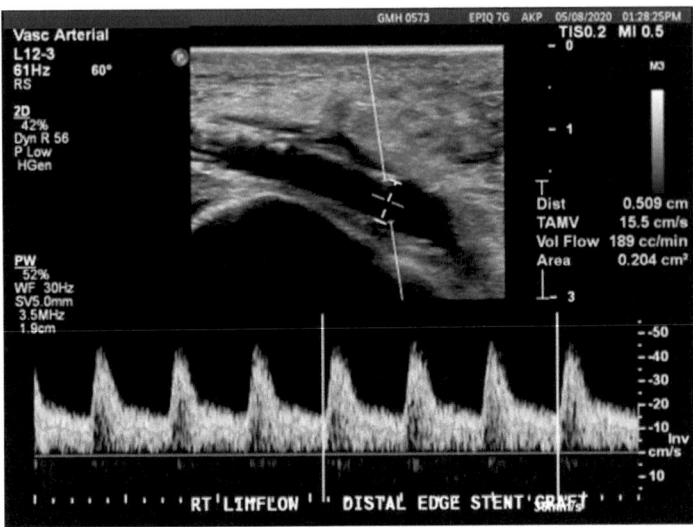

Fig. 12.1 Volume flow rate, proper technique

these branches/perforators are a pathway to divert blood flow from the pedal arch (Fig. 12.2).

(f) Toe/brachial index
- Measurement of upper extremity brachial artery systolic pressure bilaterally.
- Representative pulse volume recording (PVR tracings) at the great toe of the leg with the TADV
- Representative photoplethysmographic waveforms (PPG tracings) at the great toe of the leg with the TADV
- Toe pressures are obtained at the great toe of the leg with the TADV

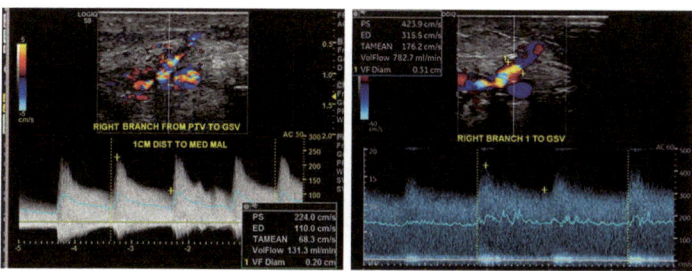

Fig. 12.2 Branches around TADV distal anastomosis

12.8 Interpretation

(a) Arterial duplex
- Degrees of stenosis for native arterial vessels proximal to the TADV circuit
  - A peak velocity ratio of 2:1 between the site of stenosis and the closest normal segment preceding it represents a ≥50% Stenosis—even moderate stenosis can threaten the long-term patency of the TADV stents.
  - A peak velocity ratio of 3:1 between the site of stenosis and the closest normal segment preceding it represents a ≥75% stenosis
  - The absence of color within the arterial segment suggests occlusion
  - A delay in systolic upstroke infers a more proximal lesion, and a decrease in diastolic flow indicates peripheral resistance and implies a distal lesion.
(b) Volume Flow Rate
- Volume flow rate normal range is 100–300 ml/min throughout the stent graft and at the lateral plantar vein level (for the first 6 months). *A long-term patent TADV circuit will fully arterialize over time, and at the 9–12 month timepoint, begin to mirror a native tibial-pedal artery with high-resistant, multiphasic waveform components.*

(c) Toe/brachial index (Fig. 12.3)
- Normal index: >0.70 equates to normal perfusion
- Abnormal index: <0.40 suggests severe disease
- Adequate digital pressures for healing wounds 55 mmHg

Fig. 12.3 TBI severity

TBI	Severity
>0.70	Normal
<0.40	Suggest Severe Disease

Circuit Maintenance and Optimization

13

Anahita Dua, Sara Rose-Sauld, and Lindsey Ferraro

13.1 Indications for Intervention Post-TADV

In a TADV patient, any changes in clinical or ultrasound indications may warrant an arteriogram. Identifying nutritive vs non-nutritive flow in the foot is critical for determining the need for possible reinterventions. Non-nutritive flow can be managed through a careful occlusion that does not impact the flow in the pedal loop. Consequently, vigilant follow-up examinations are *key* for balancing flow into the pedal loop while diverting branches. During TADV follow-up duplexes, three fundamental questions must be asked: *Is flow too high? Is flow too low? Are there stealing vessels off the arterialized vein?* Blood flow characteristic changes and TADV maturation occur rapidly in the initial weeks post-TADV, so indications for intervention of flow should be held 4–6 weeks post procedure—if not addressed during the primary procedure.

A. Dua (✉) · L. Ferraro
Division of Vascular and Endovascular Surgery, Massachusetts General Hospital/Harvard Medical School, Boston, MA, USA
e-mail: ADUA1@mgh.harvard.edu; LTFERRARO@mgh.harvard.edu

S. Rose-Sauld
Podiatry, Massachusetts General Hospital, Boston, MA, USA
e-mail: SROSE-SAULD@mgh.harvard.edu

105

- Clinical indications for intervention
  - Pain
  - Infection
  - Worsening wounds/changes in color
- Ultrasound indications for intervention
  - Marked increase or decrease in flow volume
  - Low or stagnant flow in the distal lateral plantar vein
  - Stenotic areas in inflow and/or outflow
  - Stealing branches of LPV distal to the stent
  - Maintenance of native tibial perfusion
- Significant changes in clinical or ultrasound indications warrant consideration for an arteriogram.

13.2   Flow Optimization

Nutritive vs Non-nutritive Flow in the Foot

- The venous anatomy of the foot contains multiple pathways that can divert flow proximally and away from the distal pedal loop
- Balancing the flow into the pedal loop and the diverting branches requires careful evaluation and follow-up
- In its most severe form, rapid proximal diversion into the central venous return can prevent pedal loop perfusion and decompress remaining proximal arterial perfusion (clinical arterial steal syndrome)
- Desired flow pathway: Lateral plantar vein to first metatarsal perforator to dorsal outflow (Figs. 13.1 and 13.2)
- Undesired flow pathway: Lateral plantar vein to dorsal outflow prior to reaching first metatarsal perforator (Figs. 13.1 and 13.2)

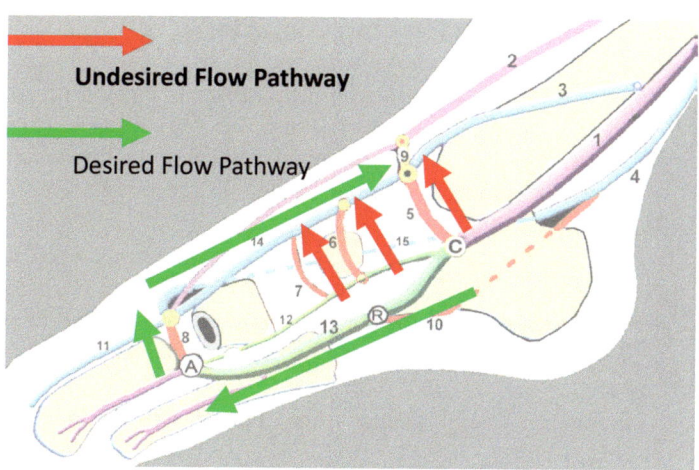

Fig. 13.1 Flow pathways, desired and undesired

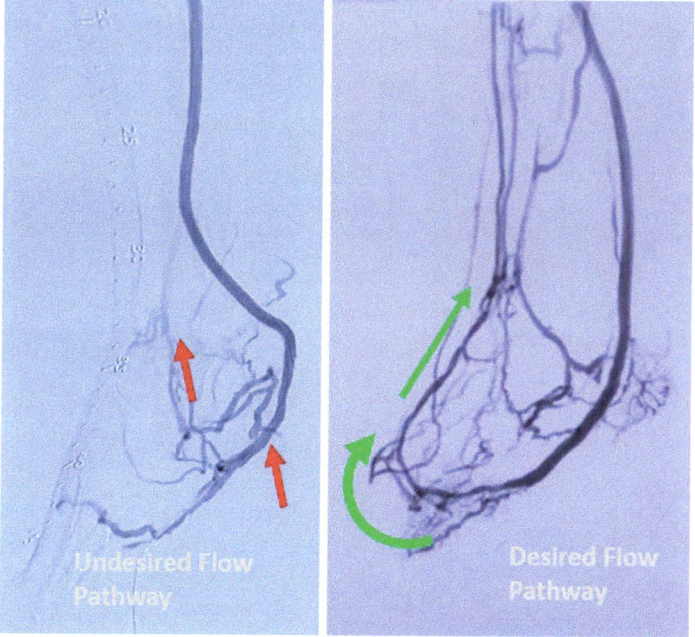

Fig. 13.2 Flow pathways

Non-nutritive Flow Imaging Characteristics

- Blood flow is diverted through a perforator or branch before reaching the distal part of the foot
- Early venous return to the popliteal level before the tibial arterial flow is complete or without similar clearance in LPV
- **What to look for:**
  - Blood flow is diverted through a perforator or branch before reaching the distal part of the foot (Fig. 13.3a)
  - Early venous return to the popliteal level before the tibial arterial flow is complete or without similar clearance in LPV
  - Failure of lateral plantar vein contrast to clear quickly (Fig. 13.3b)

    Indicates stagnant flow in the pedal loop

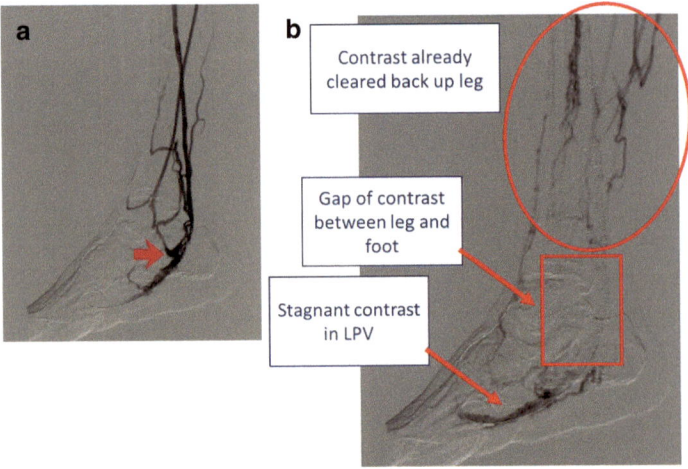

Fig. 13.3 (**a**) Blood flow diverted through perforator branch. (**b**) Stagnant flow in pedal loop

13.3   Symptoms of Non-nutritive Flow

Clinical Signs of TADV Circuit Compromise

- Foot pain after 48 h that is not localized to an open wound or ischemic tissue
- Changes in foot tissue color (mottling, cyanosis, changes from pre-op)
- Pedal loop occlusion due to low flow characteristics

13.4   Flow Management Post-TADV

- Non-nutritive flow routes can be considered for occlusion (embolization) at the primary procedure or during follow-up
- The decision to occlude a proximal branch of the lateral plantar vein is made based on the adequacy of flow through the pedal loop and maintenance of native arterial perfusion
- Care should be taken to only occlude non-nutritive outflow pathways
  - Not recommended to occlude dorsal pedal veins that function as the primary outflow
  - Ensure embolization does not impact flow in the pedal loop
- Procedural access routes that don't involve the lateral plantar vein should be considered during embolization.

13.5   Flow Management Timing

Key Indications for Intervention

- Pain—increase in level/non-resolution of pain experienced
- Infection
- Worsening wounds/changes in tissue color (cyanotic foot)

Changes in Blood Flow Characteristics and TADV Maturation Are Rapid in the Initial Weeks after TADV

- Previously closed perforators can open (failing valves)
- High flow and hemodynamic stresses may induce stenoses
- Inflow lesions not apparent during implant can worsen under high flow and result in occlusion

Timing

1. **During the primary procedure only to correct obvious sluggish or slow flow in the lateral plantar vein**
2. **During 4–6 weeks post procedure to address key indications listed above**

Example 1 Identifying venous tributaries for duplex surveillance (Fig. 13.4).

Non-nutritive flow identified via angiogram coming off the lateral plantar vein.

Case Example

- The wound at the toes did not improve pain had not improved and had increased, observed 3 months post TADV
- Arterial steal observed just distal to stent graft
- Stagnant flow observed in the lateral plantar vein
- Coil placed during follow-up procedure 3 months post TADV (Fig. 13.5)
- Pain resolved after coiling

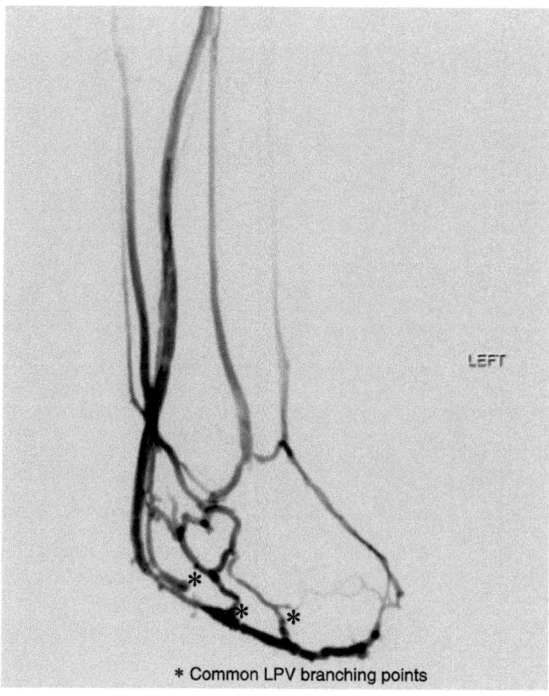

LEFT

* Common LPV branching points

Fig. 13.4 These are common branching points from the lateral plantar vein and should monitored for changes in volume flow by duplex US

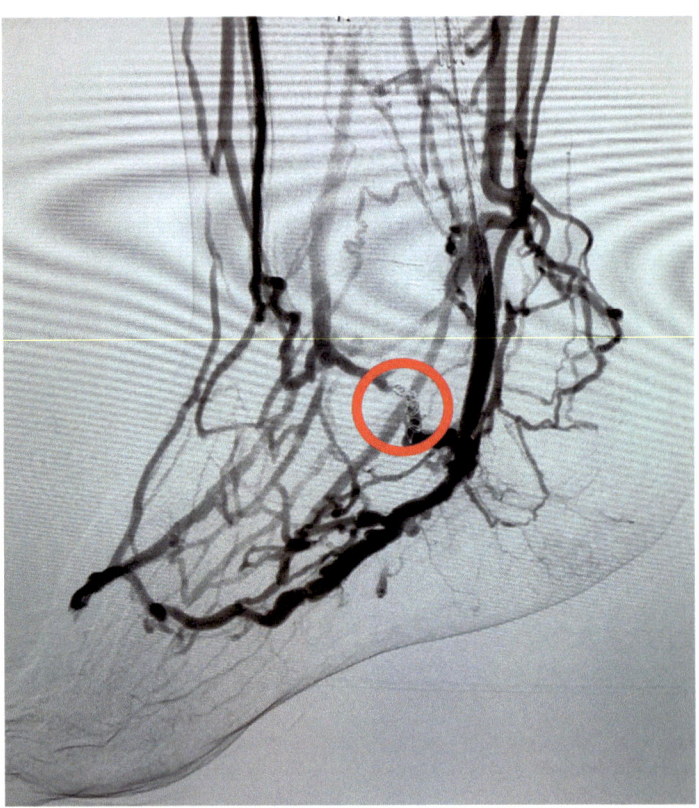

Fig. 13.5 Coil placed 3 months post-procedure

13.6 Volume Flow Interpretation

- Volume Flow (VF) rates allow us to quantify flow through fistulas by taking velocity and vessel area into consideration
- 3 issues to consider when interpreting TADV duplexes
  - Is flow too high? (Fig. 13.6)
    The flow will not perfuse small metatarsal vessels needed to reach/heal wounds

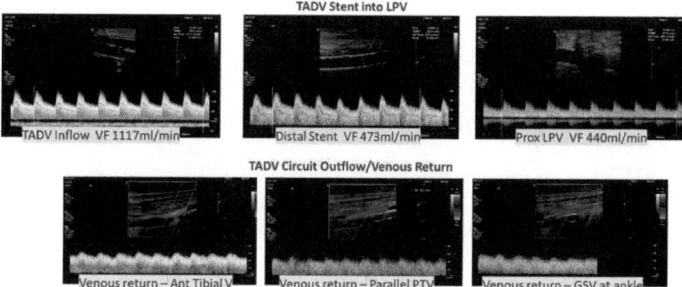

Fig. 13.6 TADV stent and circuit inflow/venous return

High VF rates throughout can signal too high of flow in the fistula.

Correlating these findings with wound healing and clinical symptoms can help determine if light compression or coiling of an outflow vein is necessary to slow the flow enough to allow adequate perfusion to the wounds. In this example, VF rates are high throughout the stent and outflow vessel.

Pulsatile venous return is also noted in multiple vessels; the greater saphenous vein (GSV), anterior tibial vein (ATV), and the parallel posterior tibial vein (PTV).

– Is flow too low? (Fig. 13.7)

Stent patency is threatened.

Native arterial stenosis, even when moderate, can threaten stent patency. Having a low threshold for re-imaging with angiography post-procedure is necessary.

Stenotic areas distal to the stent in the arterialized vein can prevent circuit maturation and wound healing when left untreated. In this example, there is a stenosis in the LPV at the proximal foot with VF rates dropping below 100 ml/min at the midfoot (<100 ml/min close to index procedure suggests future occlusion) (Fig. 13.8).

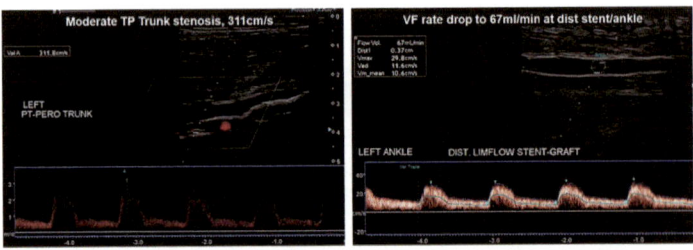

Moderate TPT stenosis resulting in a drop in VF rates to below 100ml/min at the ankle

Fig. 13.7 TPT stenosis resulting in a drop in VF rates

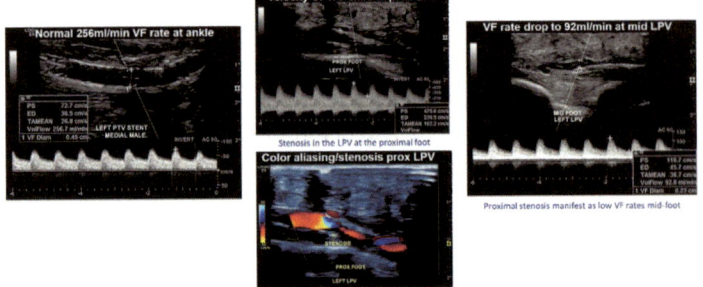

Fig. 13.8 Stenosis in the LPV at the proximal foot with VF rates dropping below 100 ml/min at the midfoot

– Are there stealing vessels off the arterialized vein? (Fig. 13.9)

> TADV circuit will likely remain patent but to no forefoot perfusion/wound-healing benefit.
>
> Stealing branches off the arterialized vein can delay circuit maturation and delay wound healing. In this example, there are normal VF rates in the stent at the ankle. A high-flow branch was noted off the LPV with a significant drop in VF rates distal to the branch. Coiling this branch will direct flow back to the LPV and will help pressurize the forefoot.

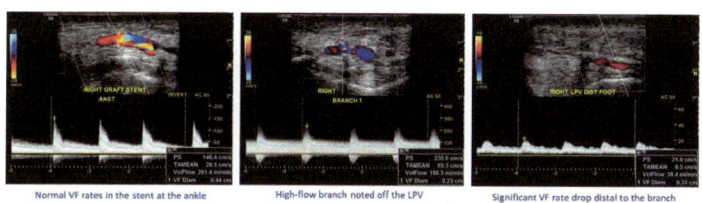

Fig. 13.9 Stealing branches off the arterialized vein

Wound Care

14

Anahita Dua, Sara Rose-Sauld,
and Lindsey Ferraro

After TADV the goal of wound care is to maintain a stable, non-infected wound until the circuit is mature. Once the circuit is mature, surgery may be performed to resect dry gangrene and optimize the patient's function. In the presence of apparent infection, debridement or minor amputations should be done only so much as to control infection. If a surgery is necessary, it is key to not debride aggressively as with typical arterialization and to avoid the use a tourniquet during amputation. *It is critical to avoid any surgery until the TADV circuit has matured, which typically takes around 3 months.* Consistency and careful management of wound care can help to prevent the need for debridement and amputation.

A. Dua (✉) · L. Ferraro
Division of Vascular Surgery, Massachusetts General Hospital/Harvard Medical School, Boston, MA, USA
e-mail: ADUA1@mgh.harvard.edu; LTFERRARO@mgh.harvard.edu

S. Rose-Sauld
Podiatry, Massachusetts General Hospital, Boston, MA, USA
e-mail: SROSE-SAULD@mgh.harvard.edu

A. Dua et al. (eds.), *The Massachusetts General Hospital Approach to Transcatheter Arterialization of the Deep Veins for Advanced Limb Salvage*, https://doi.org/10.1007/978-3-031-37510-1_14

14.1   Day 0–90 Post-TADV

- Goals: Keep dry and non-infected (prevent dry gangrene from converting to wet gangrene) until TADV has matured
- Weight-bearing:
    - When wounds present on weight-bearing surfaces
        Strict non-weight-bearing
        Consider rehab placement if this will be difficult at home
    - When small wounds on non-weight-bearing surfaces
        Protected WB, touch down weight-bearing
- Expectations:
    Highest levels of pain 3 weeks after TADV
    Dry gangrene often progresses to a degree and begins to demarcate
    The highest risk of dry gangrene converting to wet gangrene at this time
- Wound dressings: Similar to pre-op as long as no surgical events (debridement or minor amputations were done)
    Betadine-soaked gauze and dry dressing daily
    No xeroform, no hydrogels, etc.
    No compression
    If the wound becomes macerated, then BID dressing changes
- Offload bilateral heels with pillows or offloading boots while in bed to prevent heel ulcers

If clinical signs of local or systemic infection arise, or the stable wound deteriorates, debridement or minor amputation should only be performed at the level necessary for source control of the infection/wound deterioration. Amputations in the forefoot/TM level should be done without jeopardizing the pedal loop.

- Surgical debridement
    - Caution must be exercised when performing surgical debridement.
    - Newly arterialized veins in the process of maturation can bleed extensively if aggressive debridement occurs.

- Debridement earlier than 4–6 weeks of TADV must be done carefully, and remove only clear necrotic tissue.
- It is not recommended to use a tourniquet. This may cause a pedal loop occlusion
- Do not debride aggressively as is typically done after **conventional arterial revascularization**
- Do not attempt to close the wound or use a skin graft until evidence of granulation tissue is present.
- Minor amputations
  - Avoid proximal TMA, it should be mid-metatarsal
  - Do not use a tourniquet during minor amputations. This **may cause pedal loop occlusion.**
  - Be mindful of damaging the lateral plantar vein, the first metatarsal perforator, and the dorsal outflow track.
  - Primary closure is not recommended.
  - Use NPWT as a secondary dressing always when the wound shows granulation tissue. But use only low-pressure settings (50–75 mmHg), intermittent.
  - Secondary closure after wound VAC, e.g., STSG
  - Do not attempt to close the wound or use a skin graft until evidence of granulation tissue is present
  - Leave all surgical wounds open, NO SUTURES
  - Be sure all nursing and wound staff is aware NOT to perform routine debridement.
- The goal is to avoid any surgery until TADV is mature.
  - All secondary healing wounds, either after debridement or minor amputation, must be treated after a wound guideline. We recommend the international TIME (RS) wound guideline.
  - Wound management at this time is **more essential** than at the time before TADV.
    Resection of infected tissue
    No compression
    Offload the foot at all times.
    Offload heels at all times while in bed

14.2 Treatment Plan Strategy for Infected Wounds

- **Get rid of the necrotic/infected tissue**
  - Early careful surgical debridement with hydro surgery or ultrasound tools.
  - Alternatively
      Monofilament debridement
      Hydrogel, maggots
- **Treatment of the bacterial burden and biofilm**
  - Wound swab or biopsy to identify the germs
  - Use highly efficient local antiseptics (local) besides antibiotics (systemic)
- **Support growing granulation tissue**
  - If the wound is clean and if there is no major bleeding, use NPWT with low pressure (50–75 mmHg) as early as can be
  - Alternatives are advanced wound dressings
  - Tight monitoring in the hospital for 5–7 days
- **Fast and effective wound closure**
  - After the granulation tissue under NPWT reaches the wound edge and other factors support it, use STSG or other skin flaps for secondary closure.
  - Alternative: Skin substitutes
- **Offloading**

TADV and Beyond: Postoperative Care of the Patient with Forefoot Amputation

Nikolaos Zacharias

A TMA is the last hope for a diabetic patient to achieve partial limb salvage and is often difficult to heal. Based on multiple series published, approximately two-thirds of patient with TMA achieve wound healing [1–7]. Prediction of TMA wound healing is challenging most due to the multifactorial nature of critical limb threatening ischemia (CLTI), diabetes, and foot mechanics. It is even more challenging in the TADV patient.

Medical optimization of the patient with tight glucose control is crucial to the healing process of a TMA with an HbA1c target <7% [7]. Smoking cessation is equally important in order to promote wound healing and long-term patency of the deep venous arterialization (DVA).

The gait patterns of patients with partial foot amputations wearing their existing prosthesis and footwear and compared them to a nonamputee control group [8]. The gait of patients with transmetatarsal and midfoot amputations was severely

N. Zacharias (✉)
Division of Vascular and Endovascular Surgery, Department of Surgery,
Massachusetts General Hospital/Harvard Medical School,
Boston, MA, USA
e-mail: nzacharias@mgh.harvard.edu

© The Author(s), under exclusive license to Springer Nature
Switzerland AG 2023
A. Dua et al. (eds.), *The Massachusetts General Hospital Approach to Transcatheter Arterialization of the Deep Veins for Advanced Limb Salvage*, https://doi.org/10.1007/978-3-031-37510-1_15

compromised after the loss of transmetatarsal heads. Patients wearing insoles and slipper sockets maintained their center of pressure and adopted a gait pattern limiting extreme force to the residuum. The hip joints become the major sources of work during ambulation in order to compensate for the loss of ankle function [8].

Patients with TMA often develop skin breakdown that can lead to infection and higher amputation [9]. Although it is true that patients with TMA do not require as much rehabilitation as patient with a major amputation such as below or above knee amputations, when traditional footwear is used that rate of failure increases substantially [9]. A rehabilitation program focusing on protection of the residuum during the return to functional activities, and use of appropriate prosthetic devices is crucial to the long-term limb salvage and functional capacity of the patient with TMA.

Variations on Final TADV Imaging

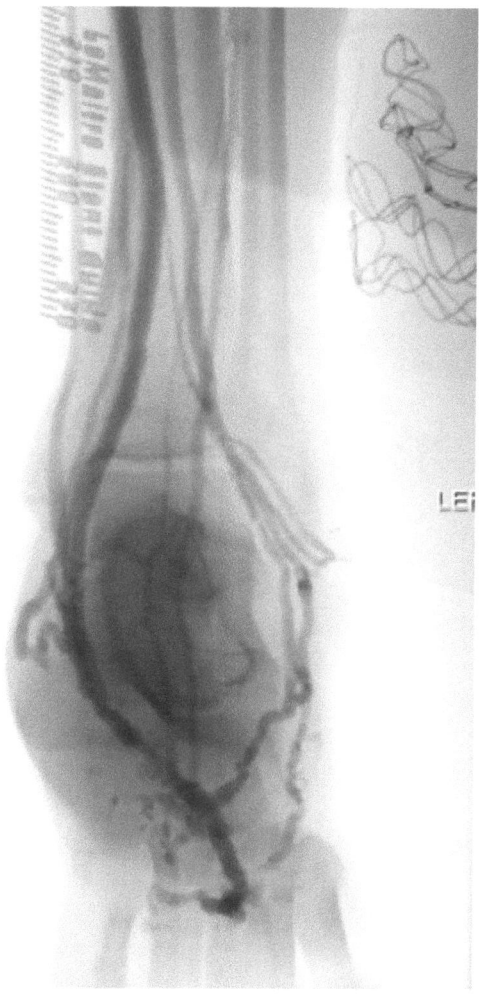

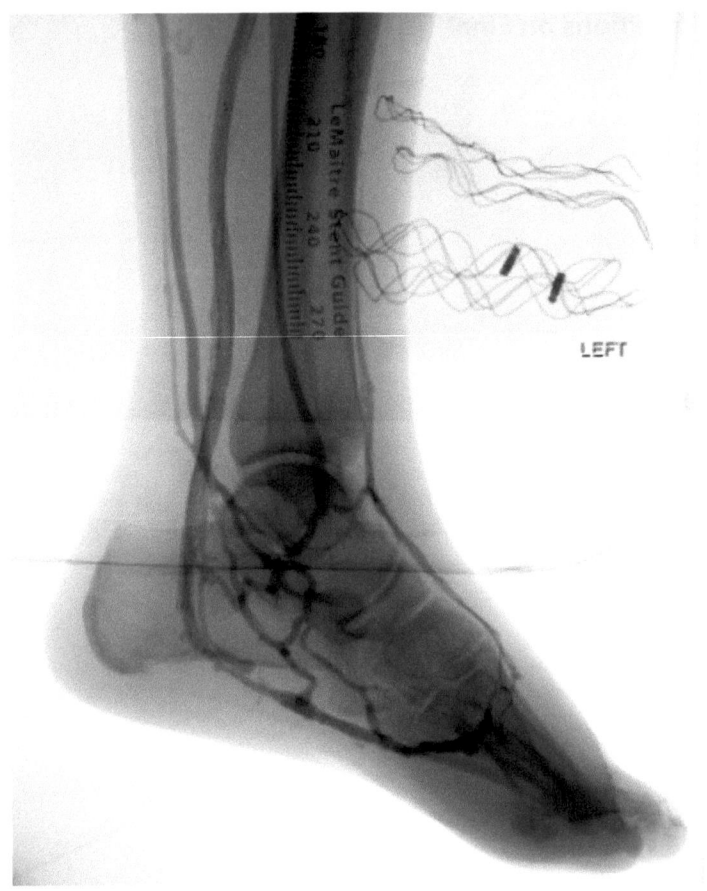

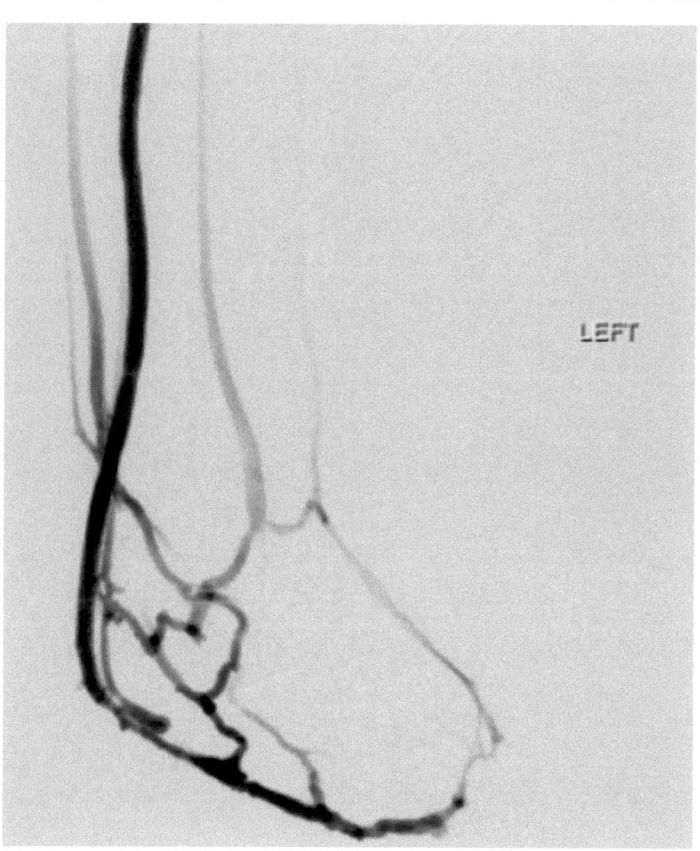

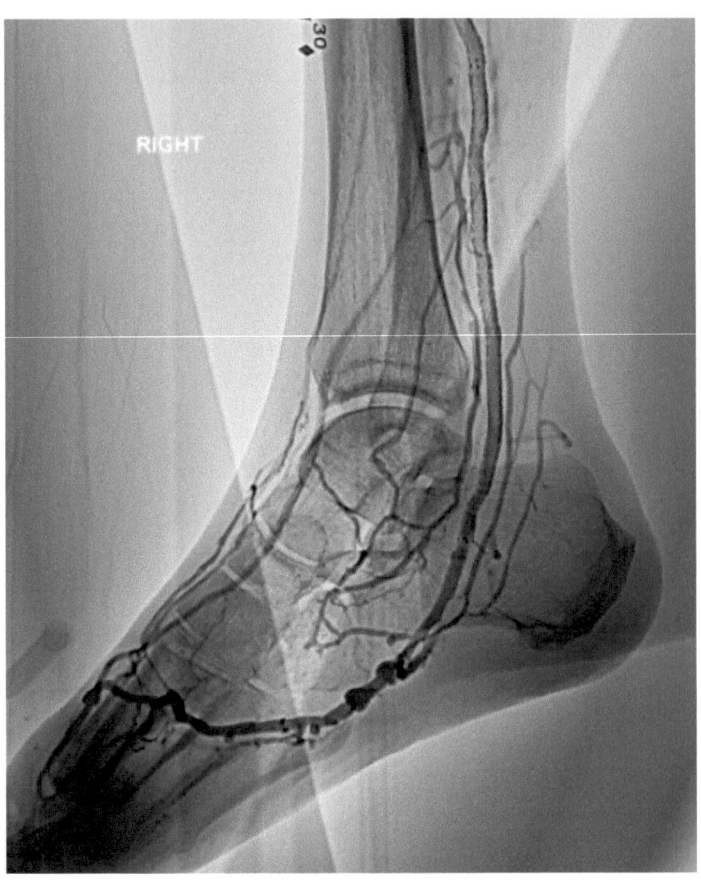

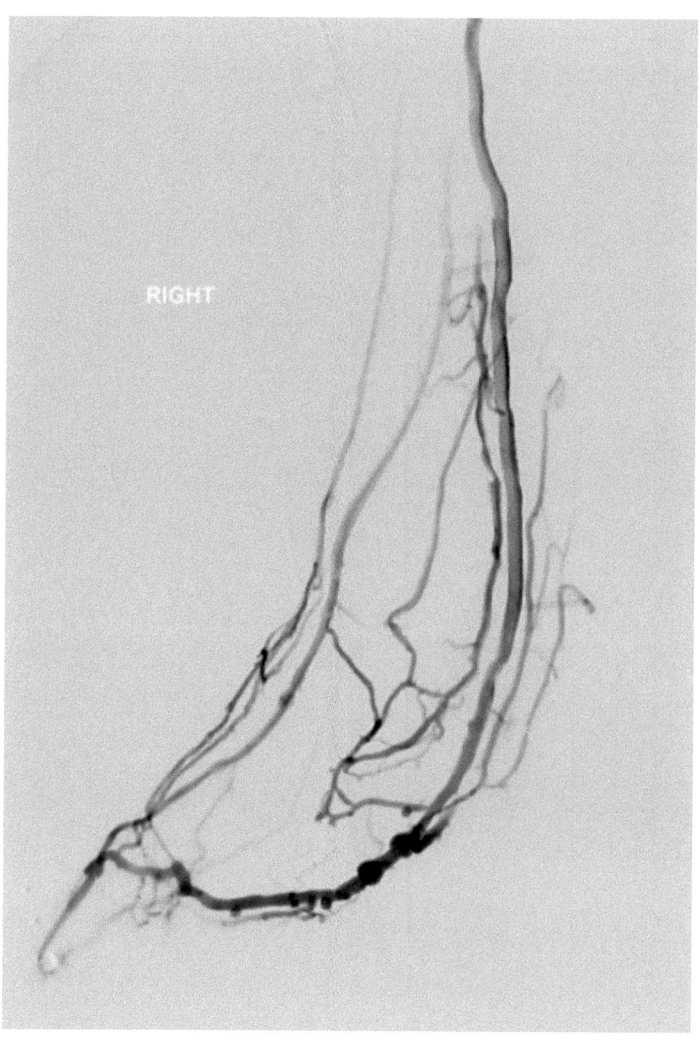

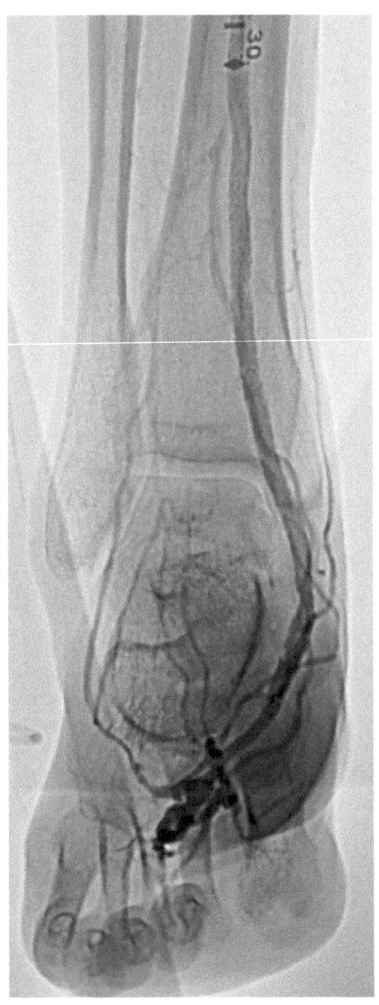

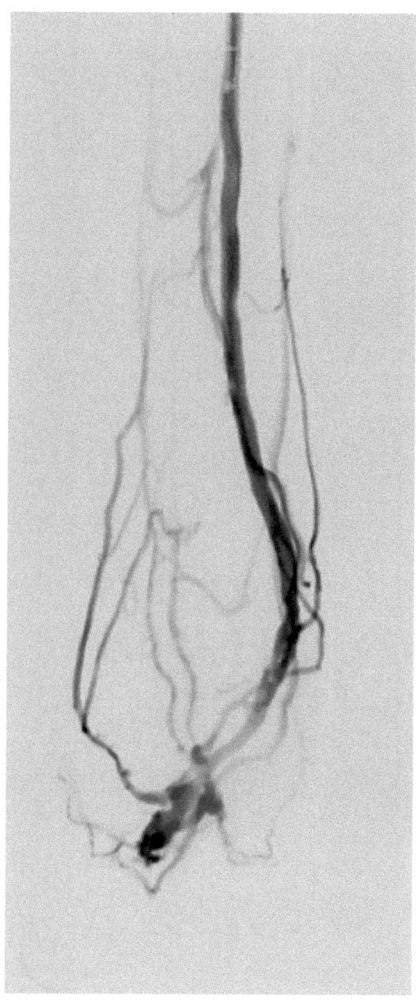

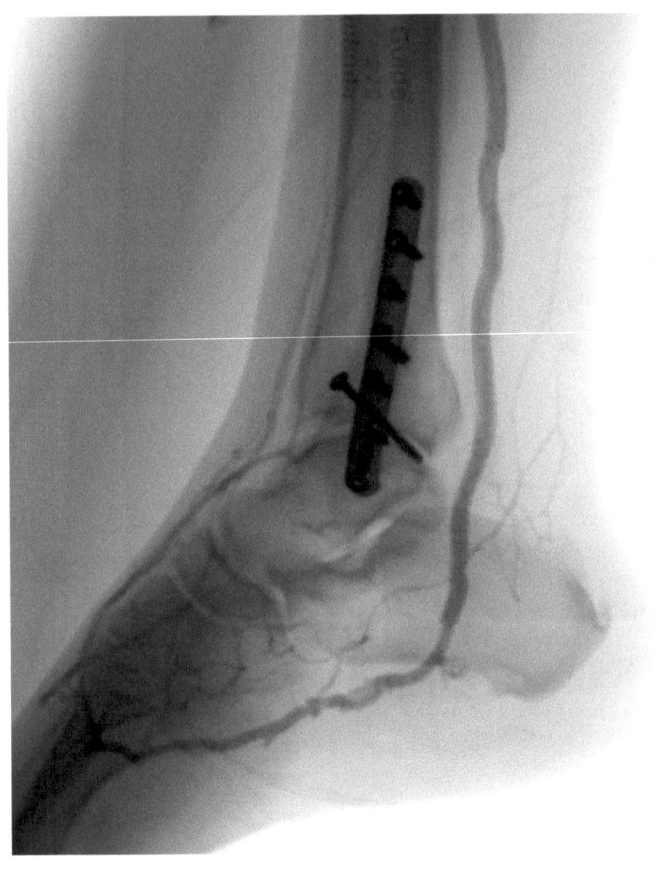

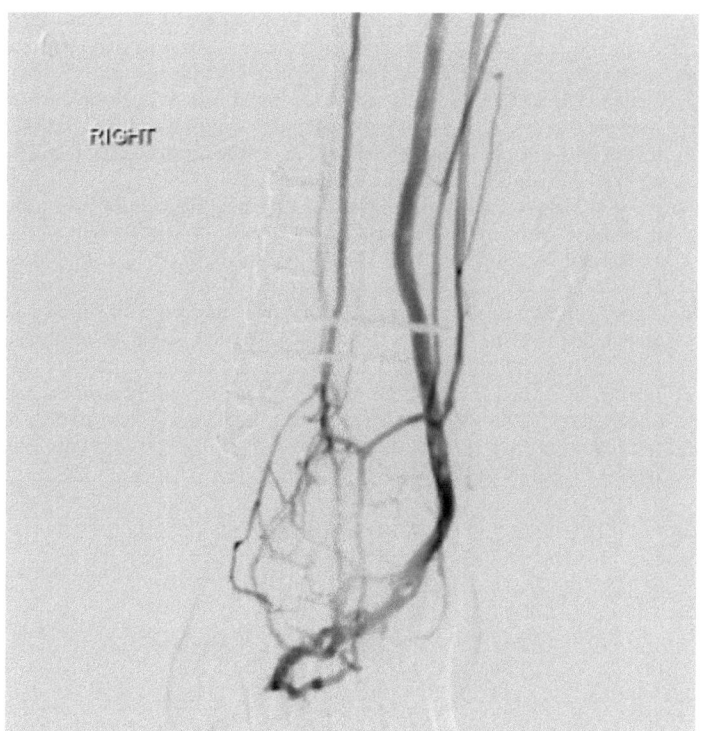

References

1. Nguyen TH, Gordon IL, Whalen D, Wilson SE. Transmetatarsal amputation: predictors of healing. Am Surg. 2006;72(10):973–7.
2. Stone PA, Back MR, Armstrong PA, et al. Midfoot amputations expand limb salvage rates for diabetic foot infections. Ann Vasc Surg. 2005;19(6):805–11.
3. Toursarkissian B, Hagino RT, Khan K, Schoofield J, Shireman PK, Harkless L. Healing of a transmetatarsal amputation in the diabetic patient: is angiography predictive? Ann Vasc Surg. 2005;19(6):769–73.
4. Landry GJ, Silverman DA, Liem TK, Mitchell EL, Moneta GL. Predictors of healing and functional outcome following transmetatarsal amputations. Arch Surg. 2011;146(9):1005–9.

5. Mwipatayi BP, Naidoo NG, Jeffrey PC, Maraspini CD, Adams MZ, Adams MZ, et al. Transmetatarsal amputation: three-year experience at Groot Schuur hospital. World J Surg. 2005;29(2):245–8.
6. Squiers JJ, Thatcher JE, Bastawros AAJ, Baxter RD, Yi F, Quan P, et al. Machine learning analysis of multispectral imaging and clinical risk factors to predict amputation wound healing. J Vasc Surg. 2022;75(1):279–85. https://doi.org/10.1016/j.jvs.2021.06.478.
7. Xiang J, Wang S, He Y, Lei X, Shanshan Z, Tang Z. Reasonable glycemic control would help healing during the treatment of diabetic foot ulcers. Diabetes Ther. 2019;10(1):95–105. https://doi.org/10.1007/s13300-018-0636-8.
8. Dillon MD, Barker TM. Comparison of gait of persons with partial foot amputation wearing prosthesis to s matched control group: observational study. J Rehabil Rees Dev. 2008;45(9):1317–34.
9. Mueller MJ, Allen BT, Sinacore DR. Incidence of skin breakdown and higher amputation after transmetatarsal amputation: implications for rehabilitation. Arch Phys Med Rehabil. 1995;76(1):50–4. https://doi.org/10.1016/s003-9993(95)80042-5.

Index

A

Access sheath, 54
Anatomical variability, 53, 54
Ancillary devices, 54, 55
Angiogram, 7–10
Anticoagulation therapy, 50, 90
Antiplatelet therapy, 50
Antithrombotic therapy, 50
Arterial catheter (ARC), 77
Arterial duplex, 100, 103
Arterial steal syndrome, 106

B

Bacterial burden and biofilm, 120

C

Calcium burden, 8, 10
Chronic kidney disease (CKD), 48
Circuit maintenance and
          optimization
    flow management, 109–112
    indications for intervention, 105,
          106
    non-nutritive flow, 108, 109
    nutritive flow, 106, 107
    volume flow interpretation,
          112–115

Circuit maturation procedures, 92
Clinical snapshot, 4
Coiling, 114
Comorbidity variability, 53, 54
Coronary artery disease (CAD), 48
Critical considerations, 4, 5
Critical limb threatening ischemia
          (CLTI), 4, 121
Crossing preparation
    ARC, 77
    arteriovenous crossing, 75
    C-arm position, 77
    conduit, 80, 81
    guidewire, 78–80
    primary alignment method, 76
    secondary alignment method,
          76, 77
    visualization and identification,
          72–74

D

Deep vein thrombosis (DVT), 39
Diabetes, 48
Diet, 46
Donor artery, 10
Dorsal venous anatomy, 58
Dual-antiplatelet therapy (DAPT),
          50

© The Editor(s) (if applicable) and The Author(s), under exclusive   133
license to Springer Nature Switzerland AG 2023
A. Dua et al. (eds.), *The Massachusetts General Hospital Approach
to Transcatheter Arterialization of the Deep Veins for Advanced Limb
Salvage*, https://doi.org/10.1007/978 3 031 37510 1

Duplex pedal mapping
    documentation, 41–43
    equipment, 38
    evaluation, 37
    indications and limitations, 38
    interpretation, 43, 44
    patient preparation, 38, 39
    procedure, 39, 40
Dyslipidemia, 49

E
Edema, 88
Exercise, 47
Expectations, 31

F
Family/support system, 31, 32
Femoral access, 71, 72
Flow management, 109, 110
Flow optimization
    non-nutritive flow, 108, 109
    nutritive flow, 106, 107
Foot infection (FI), 15, 19
Forefoot amputation, 121, 122

G
Gait patterns, 121
Gangrene, 25
Great saphenous vein, 37, 40
Guidewires, 54
Guiding catheters, 54

H
Hypertension, 48

I
Inflow vessels, 8
Ischemia, 12

L
Landing zone, 7
Lateral plantar puncture algorithm,
    70, 71
Lateral plantar veins (LPV), 40, 57
LimFlow product kit, 55
LimFlow system, 53
LimFlow VECTOR™, 82
Lower extremity, 39, 40

M
Medial marginal vein, 40
Multidisciplinary commitment, 31

N
Necrosis, 87
Necrotic/infected tissue, 120
Non-weight bearing, 27

O
Occlusions, 10
Oral factor-Xa inhibitor, 50

P
Pain management, 88
Patient compliance, 4
Patient profile, 4
Patient selection, 3–5
Pedal access and interventional
        techniques
    confirmatory venogram, 63, 65
    considerations, 63–65
    dorsal venogram of medial
            marginal vein, 66
    equipment, 63
Pedal dorsal veins, 58
Pedal loop wiring, 84, 85
Pedal plantar veins, 58
Pedal venous access

dorsal venous anatomy, 58
LPV, 57
plantar venous anatomy, 58
preoperative ultrasound, 58, 59
product recommendation, 59
Percutaneous transluminal
    angioplasty (PTA)
    balloons, 55
Peripheral artery disease (PAD), 5
Picture Archiving and
    Communications System
    (PACS), 41
Plantar venous anatomy, 58
Posterior tibial veins, 40
Postoperative care
    continuous wave doppler, 89
    edema, 88
    expectations, 88
    pain management, 88
    vascular DUS, 89
    wound care, 90
Post-procedure care planning,
    91–94
Preoperative optimization
    history, 46, 47
    medical conditions, 48–50
    physical examination, 47, 48
Prosthetic devices, 122

R
Rehabilitation, 122

S
Skin breakdown, 122
Smoking, 46
Stenosis, 103
Stent deployment, 83, 84
Stoplight approach, 7
    angiographic screening, 8–10
    wound screening
        location, 22, 23
        WIfI, 20–22

SVS, 15–20
Systemic inflammatory response
    syndrome (SIRS), 19

T
Toe/brachial index, 102
Touch weight bearing, 28
Transcatheter arterialization of the
    deep veins (TADV)
    circuit
    documentation, 100–103
    duplex ultrasound surveillance,
        97, 98
    equipment, 98
    interpretation, 103, 104
    limitations, 98
    patient preparation, 99
    procedure, 99, 100
    stages, 31–33
Transmetatarsal amputation (TMA),
    121–131
Traumatic brain injury (TBI)
    severity, 104

U
Ultimate flow, 32

V
Valve effacement, 81–83
Venous access
    crossing points and collaterals,
        68–70
    duplicate venous anatomy, 67,
        68
    lateral plantar puncture
        algorithm, 71
    spasm, 67
    target tibial, 69, 71
    thinner media layer, 67
    valves, 67
    vessel perforation, 67

Volume flow (VF), 98, 112–115
    rates, 101–103

W
Weight bearing, 118
    status, 24
Wound care, 90
    dressings, 118
    expectations, 118
    goals, 118, 119
    minor amputations, 119
    surgical debridement,
        118, 119

treatment plan strategy, 120
    weight bearing, 118
Wound closure, 120
Wound, ischemia and foot Infection
        (WIfI) classification
        system, 20–22
Wounds
    identification, 12, 14, 15, 17–19
    pre-TADV wound stability,
        23–25, 27–30
    stoplight approach
        screening, location, 22, 23
        screening, WIfI, 20, 22
Wound surveillance, 91